CARE of the POSTMENOPAUSAL PATIENT

Edited by
Frederick J. Hofmeister, M.D.

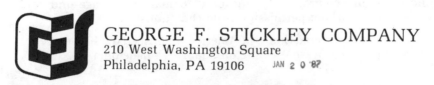
GEORGE F. STICKLEY COMPANY
210 West Washington Square
Philadelphia, PA 19106   JAN 2 0 '82

618,1
C18

Manufactured in the United States of America; Published by the George F. Stickley Company, 210 West Washington Square, Philadelphia, PA. 19106.

CARE
of the
POSTMENOPAUSAL
PATIENT

CONTENTS

Foreword... vii
F.J. Hofmeister, M.D.

Preface viii
A.F. Lash, M.D.

Evaluation of the Total Woman 1
F.J. Hofmeister, M.D.

Nutrition, Exercise and Health 11
Dorothy M. Barbo, M.D.
Florence Crawford, R.N., M.S.N.

The Estrogen-Deficient Woman 33
Alvin F. Goldfarb, M.D.

Carcinoma of the Breast............................. 47
C. Paul Hodgkinson, M.D.

The Aging Vulva...................................... 55
Eduard G. Friedrich, Jr., H.A.B., M.D., L.L.D., (Hon.)

Geriatric Gynecologic Oncology 65
C. Robert Stanhope, M.D.

Postmenopausal Bleeding 75
Murray J. Casey, M.D.

Urethrovesical Problems in Female Geriatric Patients.. 109
C. Paul Hodgkinson, M.D.

Prevention and Operative Treatment of Relaxations
and Lacerations of the Posterior Vagina
and Perineum:
    Choice of Episiotomy
    Posterior Colpoperineoplasty 115
Brooks Ranney, M.D.

Management of Pelvic Support Loss in the Geriatric
Female... 133
Wayne F. Baden, M.D.
Tom Walker, M.D.

Managing Prolapse of the Post-Hysterectomy Vagina .. 157
  Jesse A. Rust, M.D.

Care of the Dying Patient 163
  James L. Breen, M.D.
  Albert Strunk, M.D., J.D.

Index 187

FOREWORD

Newly established geriatric centers in all geographical areas and in many large and small hospitals emphasize the fact that physicians must become more aware of the problems of the aging. Certainly the gynecologist must know the requirements necessary for evaluating and caring for the geriatric woman as well as for patients of all other age groups. Many of us in gynecology have long stressed not only the need for communicating with the patient and for being a compassionate and understanding clinician, but for developing in younger physicians an interest in the health and welfare of the geriatric patient.

It must be re-emphasized that what is suggested in this book also applies to all age groups of all women. We need now to focus on some of the problems that exist in the older age group, but cancer can also be found in the very young. The youngest carcinoma of the cervix, fortunately in situ, in my own practice was discovered in a patient 16 years of age. The oldest carcinoma of the cervix was found in a patient 92 years of age. Therefore, caution, attention and individualized care are important for each patient. It is for this purpose that the contributors to this volume enthusiastically submitted material which they thought might add to the growing bank of knowledge concerning the geriatric patient.

It is in this way that we go forward to health.

F.J. Hofmeister, M.D.

PREFACE

The prolongation of life in the United States has manifoldly increased the number of geriatric patients. At the same time, families in Western society have gradually decreased their responsibility to these elderly individuals. This problem has reached that degree of magnitude that the government has now assumed an interest; the White House Conference on Aging was initiated to formulate plans for solving this problem in the United States. The vast social, cultural and economic changes occurring so rapidly in our country are being analyzed and attacked by an army of sociologists, psychologists, and welfare workers. But it is of primary importance that physicians be prepared to deal with the medical problems of this large segment of our population.

My own interest in geriatric gynecology began more than thirty years ago when large numbers of elderly women were admitted to my gynecological service at Cook County Hospital in Chicago. At that time, many birth injuries and advanced stages of neoplasms were observed. But gradually I observed in the course of private practice that as a result of better prenatal care and lay education emphasizing the importance of preventive medicine, elderly women were coming in with earlier stages of the same pathology than did those women on the charity service.

Within the same period, there began a transition from the attitude among physicians of doing nothing or very little for these patients because of age to a gradual appreciation that *age alone is not the determining factor*. There has even arisen a controversy as to whether some physicians avoid caring for elderly patients because they do not think they can accomplish as much for them as for their younger patients.

The above considerations are the motivation for this book based on rich and longterm clinical experience. The knowledge derived from the contributors' experiences suggests that regular periodic examinations may prevent—as well as recognize—initial stages of disturbed physiology or diseases of the female generative tract. When manifest pathology is present, with proper study and individual evaluation, adequate therapy can be instituted in the geriatric patient just as in the younger patient.

A.F. Lash, M.D., S.C.

CONTRIBUTORS

F.J. Hofmeister, M.D.
Clinical Professor of Obstetrics and Gynecology
Medical College of Wisconsin
Milwaukee, Wisconsin

A.F. Lash, M.D.
Professor of Obstetrics and Gynecology (Retired)
Mount Sinai Hospital
Chicago, Illinois

Dorothy M. Barbo, M.D.
Director of Gynecologic Oncology
Center for the Mature Woman
The Medical College of Pennsylvania
Philadelphia, Pennsylvania

Florence Crawford, R.N., M.S.N.
Center for the Mature Woman
The Medical College of Pennsylvania
Philadelphia, Pennsylvania

Alvin F. Goldfarb, M.D.
Department of Obstetrics and Gynecology
University of Pennsylvania School of Medicine
Philadelphia, Pennsylvania

C. Paul Hodgkinson, M.D.
Emeritus Associate
Department of Gynecology and Obstetrics
Henry Ford Hospital
Detroit, Michigan

Eduard G. Friedrich, Jr., M.D., L.L.D. (Hon.)
Professor and Chairman
Department of Obstetrics and Gynecology
University of Florida College of Medicine
Gainesville, Florida

C. Robert Stanhope, M.D.
Associate Professor of Obstetrics and Gynecology
Mayo Medical School
Rochester, Minnesota

Murray J. Casey, M.D.
Professor and Associate Chairman
Department of Obstetrics and Gynecology
University of Wisconsin Medical School;
Chief of Obstetrics and Gynecology
Director of Gynecologic Oncology
Mount Sinai Medical Center
Milwaukee, Wisconsin

Brooks Ranney, M.D.
Department of Obstetrics and Gynecology
University of South Dakota School of Medicine
Yankton, South Dakota

Wayne F. Baden, M.D.
Gynecologist, King's Daughters and the
Scott and White Memorial Hospitals
Temple, Texas

Tom Walker, M.D.
Gynecologist
King's Daughters Hospital
Temple, Texas

Jesse A. Rust, M.D.
Department of Obstetrics and Gynecology
Smith Hanna Medical Group
San Diego, California

James L. Breen, M.D.
Chairman, Department of Obstetrics and Gynecology
St. Barnabas Medical Center
Livingston, New Jersey

Albert Strunk, M.D., J.D.
Chief Resident, Department of Obstetrics and Gynecology
St. Barnabas Medical Center
Livingston, New Jersey

1

EVALUATION OF THE TOTAL WOMAN

F. J. HOFMEISTER, M.D.

When a patient is seen by a gynecologist, that patient, whether she is 14, 35, or 90 years of age should be examined in a systematic manner for total evaluation of her physical status.

It is our responsibility to evaluate the patient totally and to determine whether there is any disease or symptoms of disease present. This is not only true of the breast but of all parts of the body. As an example, routine abdominal palpation will reveal huge kidney masses, retroperitoneal masses of extensive size, and areas of severe tenderness which need additional investigation. Whenever these problems are found and are not of a gynecological nature, it is the responsibility of the gynecologist to refer the patient to the appropriate individual for further investigation, or to do appropriate laboratory investigation and then refer the patient so that proper care can be initiated.

The Importance of History Taking

Always, fundamentally and primarily important, there is the necessity of taking a complete history of the patient's past medical problems, the present complaint, when it started and what the patient's concerns are. It is especially important to document any evidence of discharges, bloody or colorless, either from the nipple area, the vaginal area, or the rectal area. If the patient is in the early 50's and still has evidence of menstrual bleeding, documentation should be made of the intervals between bleedings, the duration of the bleeding, and the quantity of blood loss. Pain associated with these episodes of bleeding should be recorded. The history should also contain documentation of problems associated with urination such as burning, pain, frequency of urination, loss of urine with walking, bending, or even while in bed. The feeling of dryness in the vagina, the feeling of pressure in the area of the vagina should be noted. The actual awareness of something protruding is important to note. All of these problems must be recorded and then investigated.

Just as this history must be accurate and complete, so the examination must be total and complete. The fact that this patient is visiting a gynecologist does not mean that all attention should be focused on the vagina. Rather, we are evaluating the *total woman*, and that means accurate blood pressure recordings, auscultation of the heart and lung area, as well as examination of the neck for palpable thyroid abnormalities and areas of glandular enlargements in the neck or supraclavicular areas. It is also advantageous to be sure there is nothing abnormal within and around the throat.

Breast Examination

No examination of any patient at any time, whether she returns in 4 or 6 months, should be done without a careful total evaluation of the breasts. The patient is told to extend her arms above her head and lean forward so that the physician can determine whether there is any evidence of areas of retraction in the breast areas. The breasts are then palpated in a circumferential manner in the sitting position both with the arms extended above the head and with the arms at the side. The patient is asked to lie down and in a supine position a careful circumferential examination of the breast is again made, with the arms at the side and with the arms extended above the head. Any painful areas, any areas of nodulation or irregularity are noted. The nipple areas are carefully examined to determine whether there is any secretion, either white

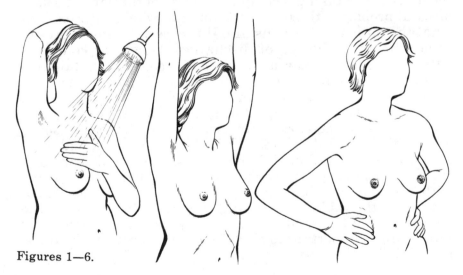

Figures 1—6.

or red. If there is any evidence of secretion, a Papanicolaou (Pap) smear is made of it and sent to the laboratory, because in my experience of evaluating patients malignant cells have been detected from areas hardly palpable, and carcinoma diagnosed from the cellular manifestation of malignancy. Another approach is to evaluate any palpable nodule to determine whether it is a firm mass or a cystic mass. If it is cystic, needle aspiration is attempted and the aspirated fluid is sent to the laboratory for evaluation. It is important to detect the very early carcinomas of the breast area; if masses are detected, verification is often extremely important. This verification is accomplished by mammography which substantiates the physician's detection; it may also eliminate the necessity for biopsy when the mammography is accurately done, interpreted, and found to be negative. If indicated, however, biopsy is essential.

While this examination is being done, the procedure is explained to the patient as well as the recommendation that on a monthly basis, preferably while in the shower or in the bathtub, she undertake breast self-examination. In fact, the patient should be given a copy of a brochure published by the American Cancer Society on How to Examine Your Breasts. (The accompanying illustrations are taken from that brochure.) First, in a circumferential manner, she is to carefully examine the breast tissue while under the shower. (See Figures 1–6.) Wet breast tissue and wet hands make for more

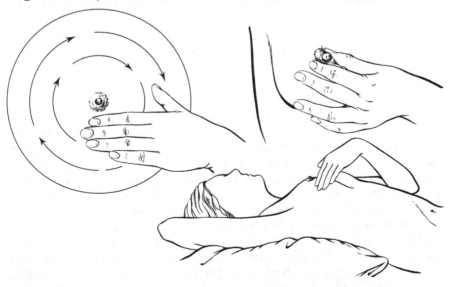

sensitive and accurate detection. This is accomplished with the arms at the side and with the arms above the head. Then it is suggested to the patient that she stand before a mirror, first with her hands on her hips, and then as shown with her hands above her head. She thus observes her own breasts to determine if there is any dimple-like retraction of the breast tissue. She then is told to lie down and again, with her arm first at her side and then above her head, circumferentially examine her breasts, the right breast with her left hand, the left breast with her right hand. Finally, she is told to attempt to express secretion from the nipples. If any is present, she should note whether it is white or red. It should be emphasized that if anything is found—a lump, a bump, a painful area, a retraction, a discharge from the nipple, either white or red, the patient should call her doctor. Her doctor should be willing to see her as quickly as possible to alleviate any fears, to determine whether masses do exist and to determine whether further investigation is necessary, either by mammography or biopsy. Communication is the key factor in helping patients detect, and thus doctors detect, early cancer or other problems, which is why the importance of explaining the procedure for breast self-examination cannot be overemphasized.

Importance of Palpation

The physician then continues with this examination by carefully palpating the abdomen for liver enlargement, abdominal masses, painful areas, pelvic masses, masses in the area of the kidneys. As indicated previously, we have found abdominal masses, not gynecological, which needed attention and were sometimes malignant because they had gone undetected prior to examination. After checking the abdomen, careful palpation and examination of the lower extremities is performed to determine whether edema is present. Following this, the patient is put in a lithotomy position and the pelvis evaluated. The labia are separated, and the patient is advised to bear down. Any protrusion of the bladder area, the area over the rectum, the uterus, or the cervix should be noted. This will give the physician an awareness of the existence of any relaxation of the female organs, any cystocele, rectocele, prolapse. The area of the Bartholin glands is checked carefully; these may have been missed because of attention to the inner aspects of the vagina rather than at the edge. Careful stripping of the urethra is important because at times the periurethral glands will be infected.

But the entire vagina is not invaded for palpation until careful inspection with a nonlubricated speculum has taken place. The speculum can be moistened with water or saline but not with a lubricant before it is inserted and the cervix exposed. The reason for avoiding palpation and lubrication is so that cellular cytology will not be interfered with. The first step after placing the speculum into position is to carefully and circumferentially collect secretion from the cervix with an Ayer spatula in both the cervical and paracervical areas. The secretion is placed on a slide then immediately prepared with fixative for a smear. There are several commercial fixatives, or a mixture of 95% alcohol and ether can be used and sent to the laboratory for evaluation of cells for malignancy. In the patient who has no uterus or who is postmenopausal, take an additional slide of the cul de sac pool area and the lateral walls to determine the maturation index; this determines the estrogen level within this patient's body. It is important to know whether there is an atrophic vagina here, whether this patient lacks hormones, whether this patient needs estrogen especially to help her have a more mature tissue in the vagina. This will help to avoid loss of urine.

It is also of great benefit to take a specimen of the secretions to determine whether there is any vaginal infection, hemophilus vaginalis, trichomoniasis, moniliasis, or gonorrhea. The vaginal infection should be detected so that accurate therapy can be initiated. The suspicion of anything of a gonorrheal nature would be best verified if culture is obtained for gonococcus.

Cervical Lesions

Any suspicious cervical lesions can be stained with the Schiller staining technique, and the areas which do not absorb the Schiller's stain can be biopsied to determine whether there is any dysplasia, carcinoma in situ or actual carcinoma. The technique becomes even more accurate if a colposcopic biopsy is performed, so this technique is recommended. If the patient has any evidence of bleeding in the postmenopausal period it is important to go one step further and do an endometrial biopsy, preferably using the Hofmeister modifications of the Novak and Randall curettes illustrated in Figure 7. They have larger apertures and are 3mm, 2mm, and 1mm in size. The Novak serrations have been changed to Haney-type serrations. All three curettes have these serrations, making for a more accurate and perfect

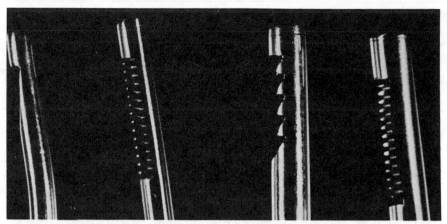

Figure 7.

method of gathering tissue. A complete circumferential evaluation of the endometrial cavity is done twice; the tissue put in formalin, sent to the laboratory, and the report forwarded rapidly after the tissue is obtained. In order to make this less distressful, there are two methods for pain relief: infiltration with 1/200,000 epinephrine and 1% xylocaine, or by dribbling in 5 cc of 4% xylocaine through the curette before this technique is performed. Allow 2 to 3 minutes after the fluid infiltrates and dribbles into the uterine cavity for the topical anesthesia to take effect. The tissue can then be collected and again sent to the laboratory. Not all patients require infiltration or intrauterine local anesthesia but many are fearful and would benefit by this approach.

Following the endometrial biopsy, a complete examination should be done in all age groups. The index finger is placed in the vagina and midfinger in the rectum, and the other hand on the abdomen. This gives the physician an opportunity to accurately determine the presence of uterine tumors, adnexal tumors, uterine immobility and cul de sac tumors. It should be explained to the patient that the vagina, uterus, and ovaries are being examined both vaginally and rectovaginally to determine the presence of any suspected disease. Sometimes there is a question about why the examination entails one finger in the rectum; the patient should be told that it is because the back part of the uterus can be felt. It is also important to note that the rectovaginal examination enables the physician to determine whether there are masses in the rectum, whether there is blood on the examining finger, and whether more extensive rectal examination is necessary because of these findings.

Before the examination is complete, careful inspection is done again (as it was before the examination started) to look for any apparently abnormal lesions on the vulva. If there is any question, a Keyes biopsy instrument may be used for biopsy. Much to the surprise of most physicians and patients, this procedure may detect an early malignancy. Early detection makes such a lesion curable with appropriate therapy.

It is part of our responsibility to examine the total woman. Has the examination been completed? A total evaluation of the physical aspects has been made, and discharges from both the breast and vagina have also been gathered for evaluation. But careful evaluation of the urine is also important. A 4+ sugar may be found unexpectedly. Evidence of infection in the urine can be found. It is important to note this as being one of the essential laboratory approaches. Finally, complete evaluation of the blood count and, where necessary, cholesterol or thyroid level should be done by appropriate laboratory testing. Only with this approach of careful *total evaluation* can the patient be assured that she has received appropriate care. When abnormalities or disease are found, appropriate care must be initiated: the following chapters contain suggestions by other gynecologists regarding their approach to some of the problems arising in the female genital organs. The emotional status of the patient must also be attended to during the evaluation, since care may be necessary for these problems.

The question frequently arises of why we do Pap tests as well. I tell all my patients of my personal belief that great progress has come to gynecology as a result of the Pap smear taken intelligently and at times indicated by the findings at examination. Cervical cancer can occur in patients of all ages, above the age of 65 as well as at the age of 16. Of all the smears done in our organization, malignancy of the cervix is detected in 1.5% of patients examined, and 20% of these are asymptomatic. Some of these patients have erratic bleeding; endometrial cancer can be detected in a small number of these patients, although endometrial biopsy is the approach of choice. In addition, inform every patient taking hormones that there should be no blown-up misconceptions about cancer related to hormones as were circulating during the past several years.

Each geriatric gynecologic patient should be given information which emphasizes the necessity for regular examinations—not at 3-year intervals but approximately every year; these examinations must be careful, total examinations including a Papanicolaou smear, and endometrial biopsies where indicated.

Finally, what number of patients come to a gynecologist in what age groups? In an evaluation of the past 1257 patients seen by me, 719 were under the age of 55, 151 patients aged 56 to 60, 126 patients 61 to 64, and 267 were over the age of 65. This shows that approximately 1/5 were over the age of 65 while 1/2 were under the age of 55. Therefore, do not neglect the geriatric patient. She too needs care, consideration, and compassion.

I feel it would be improper to close a chapter on the evaluation of the geriatric patient without reference to material which was sent for inclusion in this volume by Dr. Clarence J. Kocovsky who is an outstanding family practitioner, Chairman of the Department of Family Practice at Good Samaritan Medical Center, and involved with the care of the geriatric patient in multiple nursing homes in the Milwaukee community. It is interesting to note that during the past three years of his activity in this specific area with which he has been involved 35 years, he has found carcinoma to be a big factor among these elderly patients. He cites endometrial carcinoma, cervical carcinoma and carcinoma of the breast, which exceeded the other two types of malignancy by double the amount. Ovarian carcinoma was not as frequently found. Urinary incontinence with cystocele and urethroceles was a frequent complaint. Urethral caruncles were found on routine examination in many of the patients examined. Recorded multiple hysterectomies were performed while the patients were in the nursing home, usually for uterine prolapse and at times for uterine fibroids. Carcinoma of the vulva was rare, but all of these problems exist in nursing home patients. The significant factor is that the patient often is not carefully surveyed and must therefore be surveyed routinely to determine if there are abnormalities present. The presence of carcinoma of the breast must be investigated; in some instances the nurses on the floor have been taught to be careful and efficient examiners and have found carcinomas of the breast which would otherwise not have been detected. Also, any bleeding must be investigated by endometrial biopsy and Pap smear so that possible carcinomas of the uterus can be found.

It is important that patients, because of age, are not cast aside, according to Dr. Kocovsky. To this end, careful and complete evaluation of the patient is an extremely important factor. One final observation of importance is that he believes that estrogen therapy for people in these advanced age groups is not creating hazards but is protecting them from osteoporosis, and it continues to protect their bone structure as well as alleviate postmenopausal symptoms which include anxiety, memory loss, and extreme tension. These observations by a physician dealing with the aged patient over a period of 35 years should emphasize the statements previously made that communication and careful evaluation are essential.

2
NUTRITION, EXERCISE AND HEALTH

DOROTHY M. BARBO, M.D.
FLORENCE CRAWFORD, R.N., M.S.N.

American women reach the postmenopausal years with a third to a half of their lives ahead of them. The enjoyment of these years is at least partially dependent on good health. It is essential, therefore, that women should enter the mid-lifetime with good nutrition and in healthy physical condition. During this period, the physiologic processes of aging begin, and there is also the risk of osteoporosis, cardiovascular disease, and cancer. Though physical activity may be reduced and energy needs decline, good nutrition is still necessary to meet daily requirements and maintain health. A wide variety of foods offers the best means of obtaining balanced nutrition.

The physician should be alert for the woman with less than optimal nourishment. The malnourished are more likely to be over 75 years of age, live alone, be chronically ill, or be at the poverty level. Subclinical deficiencies may not become manifest until illness strikes and stores are then rapidly depleted. When clinical manifestations develop, or medical treatment is administered, dietary modification and/or supplementation may be needed. One should be alert to distinguish between functional symptoms of aging and disease, because the treatments are quite different. The patient needs a clear explanation of functional problems so she will not consider every symptom to be a disease, irreversible or limiting. Most functional complaints can be treated routinely.

Activity and exercise are the sum of a lifetime of behavior patterns based on interests, family desires, and physical abilities. The shift in family responsibilities for a woman may reduce energy expenditure, although she may never "retire" from some home tasks except for reasons of physical disability.

Persons who are involved with people-oriented activities tend to continue mental and physical exercise. Inactivity leads to obesity, increased cardiovascular disease, reduced pulmonary reserve, and less mental alertness. Recent studies have clearly shown that osteoporosis increases in the inactive. Thus to maintain bone strength and bone mineral content one must do muscular work which places stress on the bones. On the other hand, the wrong type of exercise could be hazardous in older years. The gynecologist, the internist and the family physician who are treating women all have the best opportunity to make recommendations for optimal nutrition and adequate exercise.

NUTRITION

Physiologic Changes and Diseases Affecting Nutrition

Aging. Aging decreases the number of metabolically active cells. Energy requirements are also reduced with decreased physical activity. After 20 years of age most people lower their basal metabolic rates by 2 percent with each decade of life. Obesity occurs when caloric intake exceeds need; it is a common condition in women. Obesity is a cause of malnutrition in the elderly and is often associated with adult onset diabetes mellitus, hypertension, heart disease, hernias, arthritis and gout.

Taste and Smell. The desire to eat is largely dependent on good taste, smells, and attractiveness of food. With increasing age, the olfactory fibers in the nasal mucosa become atrophic and decrease; loss of smell (hyposmia) is common. Absence of smell (anosmia) or impairment (dysosmia) may also develop. Taste acuity is lost because of a decreased number of taste buds in persons over sixty years of age. These individuals lose their taste for sweet and sour flavors, with less loss for the taste of salt. Atrophic taste buds cause many foods to seem bitter. Dentures which cover the palate also reduce whatever taste buds are available. Hot foods become less enjoyable. Drugs which diminish taste and smell are methimazole, penicillamine, lithium carbonate, antihistamines and antidepressants. There may be increased use of salt or sugar in an attempt to improve taste. Seasonings, vitamins and zinc sulfate may be helpful in these cases. Bad taste in the mouth is often due to dental caries or to poor oral hygiene.

Oral cavity. Disease in the oral cavity will result in marginal nutrition if food choices become limited and mostly soft foods are eaten. Of those reaching 65 years of age, 50 percent have lost all their teeth, and only 75 percent have adequate dentures. Periodontal disease occurs in 90 percent of persons over 75 years old and is a major cause of loss of teeth secondary to poor oral hygiene. Teeth darken with aging and become brittle. Caries, plaque formation, gingival recession and osteoporosis cause loosening and then tooth loss. At this point, self-image is decreased with a change in facial appearance, speech distortion, or difficulty in mastication. Bleeding gums, a common complaint, is most often due to poor oral hygiene or to ill-fitting dentures, rather than to a deficiency of vitamin C.

The tongue is essential to breathing, speaking, chewing and swallowing. Loss of tongue mobility occurs with nutritional deficiency or neoplasms. The most common site for neoplasms of the mouth is the tongue. Burning tongue (glosspyrexia) results from poor oral hygiene or vitamin deficiency. Painful tongue (glossdynia) is common in women, especially with xerostomia (loss of saliva). Xerostomia results from fewer secretory cells available with aging; this causes accelerated tooth decay, poorly fitting dentures from lack of lubricant, and difficulties in chewing or swallowing. Drugs used by the elderly which reduce saliva are antidepressants, antihistamines, antihypertensives, antipsychotic agents, decongestants, diuretics, and tranquilizers.

Good oral hygiene is essential and should be encouraged. The physician should identify those individuals who exhibit malnutrition secondary to oral problems and promptly refer them to a dentist.

Gastrointestinal.   Elderly people have dysmotility of the esophagus because of reduced peristalsis. The lower sphincter relaxes more slowly, delaying emptying, especially after stroke. Sitting down to eat permits gravity to assist with swallowing while aspiration is reduced. Hiatal hernia is common in those over 60 years of age. The stomach reduces its secretions: hypochlorhydria decreases absorption of iron, calcium, and vitamin B12. In effect, motility declines throughout the gastrointestinal tract.

Cell proliferation declines in the small intestine, with some villous atrophy and reduced functional surface. Since almost all nutrients are absorbed here, there may be a major impact on nutrition if a significant portion of functional bowel is lost. In addition, frequent use of mineral oil reduces absorption of fat-soluble vitamins.

The colon reabsorbs water and electrolytes. Aging results in loss of muscle tone, diminished peristalsis, and decreased strength of abdominal musculature, all of which are essential to elimination. Functional bowel complaints are common, with constipation present in 25 percent of this population. Constipation is defined as less than three bowel movements each week, usually stemming from poor habits and food choices. Laxative abuse is common in women. Diuretics often prescribed for the diseases of old age reduce colonic fluids. In such cases, one must be alert for diverticular disease or colonic cancer. Incontinence may occur as well with neurologic disease.

Drugs. The elderly are the single largest group of drug consumers. Residents of nursing homes are commonly prescribed 8 to 12 different medications daily. Here a careful drug history is essential. Drugs may alter taste, smell, chewing, swallowing, appetite; cause nausea and vomiting; suppress nutrient absorption; and cause constipation or diarrhea. Other medications may alter metabolism and excretion.

Surgery. Fluid and electrolyte imbalance is common from intravenous therapy in older women. If oral nutrition is not quickly reestablished, borderline deficiencies may become manifest. Prompt recognition of ileus, diarrhea, or failure to eat is essential to prevent complications which can extend the hospital stay.

Chronic illnesses. Limitation of mobility occurs in half the population over 65 years of age. Neuromuscular coordination declines. In some, physical restrictions to self-feeding occur post-stroke from residual weakness, while in others arthritis may reduce movement. Parkinson's disease causes lack of coordination. Persons using a wheelchair, cane, or walker may become exhausted from preparing a meal or just getting to the table. Whenever disease makes shopping, food preparation, eating or cleaning up difficult, additional support and planning are needed.

Radiation or chemotherapy. Radiation to the head and neck causes xerostomia and rampant dental caries. Pretreatment examination is essential and often dental extractions are necessary. Excellent oral hygiene is mandatory throughout treatment. External radiation therapy for chest, abdominal, or pelvic malignancies often results in poor appetite, with nausea and vomiting. Diarrhea due to radiation therapy also reduces absorption and causes fluid and electrolyte loss. Chemotherapy side effects are dependent on the drug given. Those which cause severe nausea and vomiting and reduce food intake for several days cause nutrition to be suboptimal. Anemia may be secondary to malnutrition or bone marrow depression.

Social Problems Affecting Nutrition

Alcohol.   This problem has increased among the elderly because of bereavement, loneliness, an impaired physical or mental condition, and loss of dentition. Food intake decreases when alcohol use is increased. One way to define alcoholism is when more money is spent on alcoholic beverages than on food. Physicians should always consider this in a malnourished person, since the resultant deficiencies reported include megaloblastic anemia and low levels of fat, protein, thiamine, folate, vitamin B12, and vitamin A.

Tobacco.   Insults and disease stemming from tobacco use are dependent on amounts consumed and duration of smoking. The oral cavity may develop leukoplakia and is at risk for cancer, as are the cardiovascular and pulmonary systems. Taste and appetite are suppressed to varying degrees.

Social and Psychological Factors.   Eating and food itself are both areas of social activity in most cultures in addition to being necessities. A drastic change in lifestyle may affect food selection and cause either rejection of food or overeating. Death of a spouse, loss of friends, new surroundings or illness may all contribute to anxiety or depression, and more recently, the decline of the extended family reduces needed support for coping with these problems. Occasionally, failure to eat may be an expression of hostility towards life or people and used to manipulate the family of the depressed person. Not eating could even signify a passive suicide intent. Conversely, a warm, friendly atmosphere stimulates the desire to eat. Those who live alone may eat while listening to the radio, TV or music. Group meals with family, friends, or at community or church functions are helpful; Meals on Wheels are another resource, particularly for the elderly or disabled. The ability of a person to care for herself, if motivated to do so, should never be underestimated or discouraged.

Financial.   Incomes usually are reduced with retirement and may then be fixed. Consequently, limitations may occur in the kind and quality of food purchased, cooking and storage facilities available, and transportation to markets. Drug expenditures dramatically reduce funds available for food in many cases, while poor choices or poor budgeting may be contributing factors. Since many senior citizen incomes fall below the poverty level, providing services especially for them should be encouraged, such as transportation, discounts, food stamps, free commodities, cooperatives and information services. Economically, it is less costly to supplement deficient diets with multivitamins and specific nutrients than to purchase multiple food items.

Nutrition, Healing, and Immunologic Defenses

There is a positive relationship between good nutrition and healing or immunocompetency. Even though there is a decline in immunologic capability with aging, it is modest. The elderly will still make protective antibodies after immunizations. Evaluation of immunocompetence may provide an indirect measure of nutritional status. Thus a healthy, well nourished person will recover more quickly from illness and the healing process is vastly improved.

Nutritional assessment. The physician or his assistant should assess each patient yearly for nutritional status, or whenever an acute illness arises. There are five major causes of malnutrition:

1. Illness interfering with food absorption or metabolism
2. Mechanical eating problems
3. Rejection of food resulting in inadequate intake of calories
4. Unbalanced intake with adequate calories
5. Excessive intake

A dietary history in the aged is most productive if it focuses on patterns and habits. Recall of the past 24 hours may be poor, and food records are often incomplete.

Weight and height are the most valuable assessments when they are compared with previous recordings. Loss of cutaneous fat, muscle wasting, or skin changes are other diagnostic clues. Laboratory tests to screen for deficiencies include hemoglobin, total lymphocyte count, and serum albumin. Other testing is specific and should be ordered only when a particular deficiency is suspected.

Nutritional Needs of the Elderly

Decreased energy requirements are primarily due to reduced physical activity, with a lesser reduction from slowed metabolic rate and fewer functioning cells. Individual requirements vary widely depending on body size and activity. Values have been established for younger age groups and for those over 55 years of age. These values, however, do not allow for disease, medications, or activity level.

Caloric needs for older adults of both sexes are:

Age	Range	Mean
51–75	1400–2200/day	1800
76 and over	1200–2000/day	1600

Caloric distribution for older women is:

Carbohydrates	50–55%
Fat	30–35%
Protein	13–30%

Reduction of caloric intake in aging years necessitates greater care in food selection. The most common deficiencies we encounter are in calories, calcium, iron, thiamine, and riboflavin.

Complex carbohydrates are the most desirable, because they add fiber and nutrients compared to refined sugars. They are also important metabolically in preventing ketosis.

Dietary fat is a source of essential fatty acids and fat-soluble vitamins. Fat delays digestion and absorption; it enhances the taste of food. Lower fat diets contribute to a sense of well-being, so the use of polyunsaturated oils should be encouraged.

Protein requirements for older women have not been established. However, surgery, injury, illness, or infection increase the need for amino nitrogen to aid healing.

Vitamins have been evaluated in many groups of our elderly population. Lower values are associated with daily caloric intake below 1500 in residents of nursing homes, when concurrent diseases interfere with nutrition, and medications reduce absorption or storage. The most common deficiencies are thiamine and riboflavin, with the intake of vitamins A and C frequently borderline. Low vitamin D levels occur mainly in housebound women who have almost no exposure to sunlight or when hepatic or renal disease impairs conversion. Only 15 minutes of exposure to sunlight daily is required for most to permit the body to make vitamin D. Fortunately, today commercial milk sold in the United States is enriched with vitamin D.

Excesses do occur with our modern megavitamin cultism; the elderly and the ill are often victims of hardsell quackery and promises of cure. Generally, a daily multivitamin tablet containing the RDA is sufficient for supplementation of the diet.

Minerals. *Calcium* needs continue throughout life. The RDA for calcium are listed at 800 mg for women. Many in the nutrition field now recommend 1000 mg daily in the premenopausal years and 1200 to 1500 mg daily after the menopause. Yet the average calcium intake of American women is still only 400 to 500 mg per day. It is not surprising, then, that skeletal weights decrease when intake is inadequate and that less absorption of calcium occurs, partially due to lower estrogen levels. The Ten-State Survey found this bone loss to be independent of economic status. As bone remodeling takes place, there is inadequate calcium for replacement, a silent loss which continues at a rate of 1 percent per year. Evidence now suggests that a calcium-rich diet can help prevent osteoporosis. Exercise is also essential to stress bones and challenge them to replace calcium. Exogenous estrogen replacement can increase absorption in the intestine and stimulate bone replacement.

A calcium-rich diet is ideal. A quart of milk daily largely meets the adult human need for calcium. Other good sources are milk products as cheese, yogurt and ice cream. Consuming low-fat milk or cheese will reduce calories. See Table 1 for a list of sources of calcium-rich food.

If a woman has a lactose intolerance, dislikes milk products or is concerned about her calorie intake, supplemental oral calcium should be prescribed. The best type of absorbable mineral is calcium carbonate or oyster-shell calcium (41 percent elemental form). This should be taken on an empty stomach or at bedtime to avoid combining it with dietary fiber which is then lost in excretion. Constipation may occur initially; fruits, vegetables and increased fluids will help to compensate for this. Some tablets also contain vitamin D. Oral mineral supplements are no more expensive than milk if generic brands are purchased.

Potassium is essential for patients taking diuretics or cardiac medications. It is found in fresh citrus fruits and some vegetables. Excretion of potassium may be reduced in renal disease.

Magnesium is essential in key enzymatic reactions, for neuromuscular transmissions and activity. Excessive magnesium antacids or laxatives coupled with reduced renal function can lead to toxicity, however. Deficiencies can occur with

TABLE 1

Food	Amount	Calcium (mg)	Calories
CHEESE			
Ricotta (made from skim milk)	1 cup	669	340
Parmesan (approx. 1/4 cup)	1 ounce	390	130
Gruyere	1 ounce	287	117
Swiss	1 ounce	272	105
Provolone	1 ounce	214	100
Mozzarella (made from skim milk)	1 ounce	207	80
Cheddar	1 ounce	204	115
American	1 ounce	174	105
American cheese spread	1 ounce	159	80
Low-fat cottage cheese-1%	1 cup	138	165
MILK/CREAM PRODUCTS			
Nonfat instant dry milk	1 cup	837	245
Thick vanilla milkshake	11 oz	457	350
Yogurt (nonfat milk)	8 oz	452	125
Yogurt-plain	8 oz	415	145
Yogurt-fruit	8 oz	343	230
Nonfat skim milk	8 oz	302	85
1% fat milk	8 oz	300	90
2% fat milk	8 oz	297	120
Whole milk	8 oz	291	150
Buttermilk	8 oz	285	100
Sour cream	8 oz	268	495
Pudding (cooked from mix using milk)	8 oz	265	320
Frozen custard	8 oz	236	375
Ice cream (11% milk fat)	8 oz	176	270
Light cream for coffee	1 tbsp	14	30
Butter	1 tbsp	3	100
FISH			
Sardines with bones	3 oz	372	175
Oysters (13-19 medium)	1 cup	226	160
Salmon (do not discard bones)	3 oz	167	120
Shrimp	3 oz	98	100
Tuna (in oil)	3 oz	7	170
FRUITS			
Rhubarb with sugar	1 cup	211	380
Orange sections-no membranes	1 cup	74	90
Whole orange-2⅝" diameter	1	54	68
Dates	10	47	220
Blackberries	1 cup	46	85
GRAINS/BREADS			
Homemade macaroni & cheese	1 cup	362	430
Canned macaroni and cheese	1 cup	199	230

Medical College of Pennsylvania, The Center for the Mature Woman

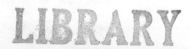

TABLE 1 (continued)

Food	Amount	Calcium (mg)	Calories
GRAINS/BREADS (contd)			
Waffle (mix, egg and milk)	one	179	205
Farina	1 cup	147	105
Beans with tomato sauce	1 cup	138	310
Homemade spaghetti (enriched with tomato sauce & meatballs)	1 cup	124	330
Corn muffin (made with egg & milk)	one	96	130
Bread (plain white)	1 slice	21	70
VEGETABLES			
Collard greens	1 cup	357	65
Turnip greens-fresh	1 cup	252	30
-frozen	1 cup	195	40
White mustard cabbage	1 cup	252	25
Kale	1 cup	206	45
Mustard greens	1 cup	193	30
Spinach (raw)	1 cup	167	40
Beet greens	1 cup	144	25
Broccoli (include stalks)	1 cup	136	40
Sauerkraut	1 cup	85	40
Cooked cabbage (shredding, chopping decreases calcium)	1 cup	64	30
Fresh green or yellow beans	1 cup	63	30
Frozen	1 cup	54	50
Carrots-crosswise cuts	1 cup	51	50
Raw 7½″ x 1⅛″	one	27	30
MISCELLANEOUS			
Almonds	1 cup	304	775
Pizza-cheese	¼ of 14″ pie	290	370
White sauce	1 cup	288	405
Cream of mushroom soup	1 cup	191	215
Cream of chicken soup	1 cup	172	180
Cream of tomato soup	1 cup	168	175
Blackstrap molasses (3rd extraction)	1 tbsp.	137	45
Tofu	3½ oz.	128	72
Chicken àla King-homemade	1 cup	127	470
Custard pie	⅐ of 9″ pie	125	285
Candy bar-sweet milk chocolate	one bar	54	126
Egg (boiled)	one	28	80
Chicken	3 oz	9	160
Hamburger	3 oz	9	185
Peanut butter	1 tbsp	9	95
Fish-most kinds without bones	3 oz	25	
Meat-most kinds lean	3 oz	9	

Medical College of Pennsylvania, The Center for the Mature Woman chronic alcoholism, total parenteral nutrition, chronic renal disease, or gastrointestinal problems, and some endocrine diseases. Meats are a rich source of magnesium.

Phosphorus has an inverse relationship to serum calcium. It is abundant in red meats, colas and "junk foods." Excesses occur more commonly than do deficiencies.

Iron demands are less when menstruation ceases, but it is still essential for hemoglobin, myoglobin and enzyme productivity. Women may develop anemia from low intake, renal disease, or gastrointestinal bleeding. Elderly women need 10 mg per day.

Copper is essential for proper utilization of iron, hemesynthesis, connective tissue metabolism, and enzymatic systems. It can be lost with prolonged diarrhea. Copper and zinc also promote taste sensitivity.

Zinc is needed for optimal utilization of amino acids and carbohydrates. Deficiencies may be manifested by impaired wound healing or poor immunologic response. Excessive losses may occur from the intestine.

Fluorine is important in tooth development and helps prevent dental caries. It is incorporated into bone and may play a role in resistance to osteoporosis. This trace mineral is toxic when excessive amounts are taken which are manifested by nausea or vomiting, fasciitis, optic neuritis, fluorosis or spinal stenosis. In drug form, it should be given only under the careful supervision of a knowledgeable physician for a specific time period.

Water is required every day to replace losses. The usual turnover rate is 6 percent of the total body water. Water assists with absorption of nutrients and keeps fecal contents soft to prevent constipation. The thirst center is less sensitive in older adults. Patients may limit their intake to reduce frequency of voiding or incontinence. Generally five to six glasses daily are needed, depending on body size and activity.

Fiber from plants includes lignin, cellulose, hemi-cellular and pectin materials. Six to ten grams should be eaten daily. Fiber, bulk and fluids are all related to transit time in the colon. The benefits are reduced absorption of fats, and glucose is combined with fiber and excreted. Oral glucose tolerance curves may improve. Drug levels may also be reduced as digoxin. Good sources of fiber are whole grain cereals or flour, legumes as peas or beans, cruciferous vegetables (cabbage, broccoli, cauliflower, kohlrabi), and other vegetables and fruits. Commercial products of lactalase are available for those with chronic constipation, diverticulosis, or other bowel diseases.

Suggestions to Improve Nutrition

- *Avoid obesity.* It limits mobility and aggravates diabetes, hypertension and arthritis. Reduce the empty calories of refined sugars. Increase the use of nutrient-dense foods such as fruits, vegetables, and grains.
- *Reduce fat intake to 30 percent of calories.* Especially reduce cholesterol-rich foods. This helps to avoid excessive weight.
- *Meals should be smaller* and regular with food chewed thoroughly. Avoid foods which cause indigestion.
- *Increase intake of fiber* in whole grain cereals, breads, fruits and vegetables.
- *Include foods rich in vitamin A or C*—dark green or yellow vegetables and fruits.
- *Decrease salt intake.* Recommend use of other spices, seasonings and lemon to improve taste.
- *Milk products,* especially low-fat, should be included in 2–3 servings daily to ensure adequate calcium. Oral calcium supplements may be added to reach a total of 1200 to 1500 mg daily.
- *Be moderate* in consumption of salt-cured, smoked, or nitrite-cured foods.
- *Encourage eating meals with other people,* at least once daily. Make mealtime a pleasant experience.
- *Recommend food alternatives* and community resources for women with low income.
- *Make positive therapeutic recommendations.* Involve nurses, dietitians, and family members to implement suggestions.

EXERCISE

Benefits

Weight control is desired by most women because it enhances self-image and esteem. The risks of cancer, cardiovascular disease, and arthritis are reduced as well. But to lose one pound requires a reduction of 3500 calories. Therefore eating 500 calories less every day for a week results in the loss of only a pound. However, weight reduction is hastened by adding exercise. With a program of regular exercise only, 15 to 20 pounds may be lost in a year *without dieting.* The slower metabolism of older years makes weight loss more difficult, so that regular activity is sometimes the only means of lowering the body's inherently desired weight level.

Mental health improves with physical activity. It reduces tension, anger, frustration, and there is enhancement of self-esteem with a more positive outlook.

Cardiovascular benefits would include a stronger heart, lower blood pressure, less risk of heart attack and stroke; lipid levels may decline and HDL rise.

The musculoskeletal system improves by increasing lean muscle as fat is lost. As tone is improved so is bodily appearance. Coordination may be better. Joint stiffness decreases and flexibility improves so that aches and pains are often relieved. Major muscles of the shoulders, arms, back, and legs should be involved. Exercise emphasizing smooth rhythmic motion with stress to bone is desirable.

Osteoporosis risk and fractures can be decreased by increasing bone work or weight-bearing. This stimulates osteoblastic activity and deposition of calcium for bone strength. Vigorous exercise should be promoted in young women to assist them in acquiring bone calcium content before the age of 35 years, after which a decline begins. However, women need consistent exercise throughout life in order to maintain bone strength. Women who begin the postmenopausal years with a high bone mineral content are at less risk, but must still continue exercising, with adjustments for medical conditions, to maintain bone strength.

The gastrointestinal tract responds to exercise by a more rapid transit time and better elimination of stool and flatus.

Sleep disorders are common in the elderly. Muscular work on a regular basis tires the body. But exercise should be avoided just prior to bedtime since it elevates norepinephrine and serotonin which prevent sleep, although the elevation of these chemicals may relieve depression.

Exercise history. The history should be specific for the types of exercise enjoyed or disliked, skills developed, and the time spent exercising each day. The interests of husband and family are important. What equipment or facilities are already available? Does she have a membership in a club, or YWCA, one convenient to home or work?

Medical Examination. A woman in good health with a normal physical examination and negative history may be encouraged to begin a basic exercise program. Limiting factors are coronary artery disease, angina, severe hypertension, peripheral vascular disease, restrictive pulmonary pathology, or orthopedic problems.

Recommendations

Women need specific recommendations and guidelines about the various types and amounts of exercise. (This effectively acts as a prescription.) To maintain physical fitness the cardiovascular system must be regularly exercised to near maximum capacity by working the body muscles. This increased demand of oxygen stimulates the cardiovascular and pulmonary systems to increase work-loads, which can be measured as maximum oxygen uptake as a result of increasing heart rate from its reserve. To improve fitness, at least 60 percent of maximum oxygen uptake must be attained and sustained for 20 minutes. A woman can improve these values by regular endurance training. Fitness is achieved when the heart rate decreases by at least 30 beats per minute within the first 60 seconds after cessation of maximum exercise sustained for at least 2 minutes. Anaerobic threshholds can be improved by challenge with interval timing (alternating fast and slow periods to allow recovery). The older the woman, the more slowly limits should be increased. A person may measure her own improvement by taking her pulse (carotid is easiest) after 20 minutes of sustained exercise which raises the pulse rate to a target zone (70–85 percent of heart capacity from prepared charts). Regardless of the type of activity chosen, one should begin slowly with a 5-minute warm-up and end with an equal slow-down time. This helps prevent cardiovascular overload from sudden cessation. Pulse rates should be maintained for 20 minutes. Excessive work will not improve performance and may risk damage to joints and muscles. Usually cardiovascular fitness furthers skeletal fitness, since muscles of the upper and lower extremities are involved in the work.

Types of Exercise for Older Patients

Aerobics and stretching will tone muscles and limber up

Figure 1. Isotonic Exercises.

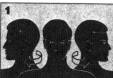

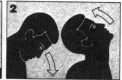

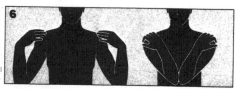

1. Stand or sit erect with chin tucked in close to chest. Turn head slowly to right, trying to bring your chin over your right shoulder. Hold for three seconds; rotate head back to center position. Pause. Repeat in opposite direction. Repeat entire sequence 5 times.

2. Push chin downward, trying to touch it to your chest, without causing too much strain. Pause. Slowly lift head backward as far as possible without straining. Pause. Repeat 5 times.

6. Upper back stretch: Sit erect. Place hands on shoulders. Try to cross your elbows by bringing your right arm to the left and left arm to the right, until you feel the stretch across your upper back. Return to starting position, drop your hands and relax. Repeat 10 times.

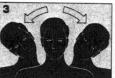

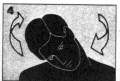

3. Bend your head slowly to the right, trying to bring your right ear to your right shoulder. Pause. Return slowly to center position. Pause. Repeat in opposite direction. Repeat sequence 5 times.

4. Roll your head clockwise in as wide a circle as possible (up, to the right, down, to the left) for three complete circles. Do the same in the opposite direction (counterclockwise). Pause. Repeat sequence 3 times.

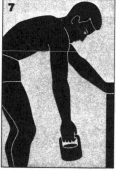

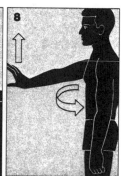

7. Pendular exercise: Hold a 1- to 2-pound weight in your hand. Bending knees slightly, bend forward at waist and hold onto a table with other hand. Allow your arm to dangle freely. (A) Swing arm laterally across body (to the right and left) for 1 minute, *keeping your elbow perfectly straight.* (B) Then swing arm backward and forward for 1 minute. (C) Then swing arm in a gradually increasing circle clockwise for 1 minute. (D) and finally, repeat (C) counterclockwise.

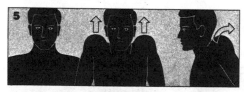

5. Shoulder shrug: Stand erect, arms held loosely at sides. Breathe deeply as you lift your shoulders first as high and then as far back as they will move. Breathe out as you lower your shoulders to the starting position and relax. Repeat 20 times, at least twice a day. Build up this routine to 50 times, twice a day.

8. Climbing-the-wall-exercise: Face the wall. Keeping your elbow straight, "walk" your fingers up the wall as high as you can go. (Do not shrug or hunch your shoulder or tilt the upper half of your body.) Repeat 10 times, each time trying to "walk" a little higher. Turn your body slightly and repeat 10 times. Continue gradually turning your body and repeating the exercise until you are at a right angle to the wall. Perform this exercise for 10 minutes, 2 or 3 times a day.

Figure 1. Isometric Exercises (continued)

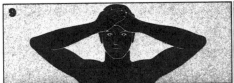

9. <u>Resisted flexion (neck)</u>: Stand or sit erect. Place one hand on top of the other on your forehead. Push your head forward against the heel of your hand, *without* moving your head. Hold for a count of 10 (approx. 7 seconds). Relax. Repeat 3 times.

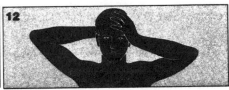

12. <u>Resisted rotation:</u> Stand or sit erect. Place your right hand on right temple and your left hand on the left side of the back of your head (your hands should be diagonally opposite). Attempt to look over your right shoulder, resisting the movement of your head with your hands. Hold for a count of 10 (approx. 7 seconds). Relax. Repeat in opposite direction, with left hand on left temple, etc. Relax. Repeat sequence 3 times.

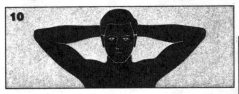

10. <u>Resisted extension (neck)</u>: Stand or sit erect. Clasp your hands behind your head—not your neck. Push your head backward against the resisting hands, *without* moving your head. Hold for a count of 10 (approx. 7 seconds). Relax. Repeat 3 times.

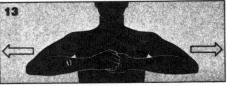

13. <u>Resisted flexion (shoulder)</u>: Stand or sit erect. Raise both forearms in front of body, parallel to ground, with elbows bent. Intertwine fingers and pull. Hold for a count of 7 (approx. 5 seconds). Relax. Repeat 3 times.

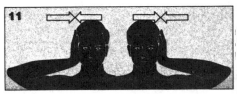

11. <u>Resisted side-bend:</u> Stand or sit erect. Place your right hand on the right side of your face. Push your head sideward against your hand. *without* moving your head. Hold for a count of 10 (approx. 7 seconds). Relax. Repeat in opposite direction (i.e., left hand on left side of face). Repeat sequence 3 times.

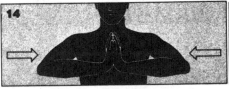

14. <u>Resisted extension (shoulder)</u>: Stand or sit erect. Raise both forearms in front of body, parallel to ground, with elbows bent. Place both palms flat against each other and press. Hold for a count of 7 (approx. 5 seconds). Relax. Repeat 3 times.

joints. A warm-up and slow-up regimen is also recommended with this type. However, cardiovascular fitness is usually not attained with this alone unless more strenuous muscle exercises are included.

Walking briskly with arms swinging freely is an excellent method for beginners and older patients. It is less stressful to joints than running or jogging, especially for those over 50 years of age. A daily walk over a measured distance to work, shop or with friends is suggested. Stationary jogging on a small trampoline may be done in any weather or at any time with little stress to joints. (However, here balance must be good.)

Swimming exercises the body symmetrically and tones up arms, shoulders, waistline, hips, and legs. It is a wise choice for women with orthopedic problems or physical handicaps, since no weight-bearing is required. Water temperature is important—chilling is to be avoided as well as overheating. Unless a progressively vigorous swimming program is carried out, no cardiovascular benefits are obtained. Unfortunately, the availability of pools and the right season may limit this activity for older people.

A stationary bicycle requires no weight-bearing or balancing. It may be done at any convenient time of day or in any weather. Equipment need not be expensive, but it should have the ability to increase resistance and measure distance. A properly fitting seat is essential; various sizes and shapes are available, although the height may need adjusting. The model purchased should be tried out beforehand to assure comfort and noise level. Exercising to music or when watching television makes it more enjoyable.

Tennis, raquetball, or squash may be of interest to those who have these skills and have enjoyed it previously. However, an elderly beginner may find it stressful to the joints.

Golf offers a good opportunity to walk, although the weight of the equipment may be excessive. On the other hand, golf alone may not provide cardiovascular fitness.

Skiing is excellent exercise for the experienced. An elderly beginner may be more likely to take to cross-country skiing, which can also be done indoors with equipment which simulates it. This is probably one of the best all-around methods available, and most challenging.

Specific Exercises for Specific Problems

Neck, shoulders, back, and joints become achy and painful

from stress, work, and arthritis. Relief may be obtained by using simple specific exercises for each area, after which comfort, flexibility as well as posture should improve.

Kyphosis from osteoporosis may be partially prevented by good posture and by strengthening para-vertebral muscles. Muscle exercises for this area also challenge spinal bones to osteoblastic activity and calcium deposition (see Figure 2).

Low back pain is common in women of all ages. Poor posture, improper lifting posture, and poor back care are major factors. Corrective exercises may be prescribed after possible pathology has been excluded. These exercises are shown in Figure 3.

Activity for the disabled should be strongly encouraged within their limitations or abilities. Do not underestimate them! Swimming is one of the best forms of exercise for women with disabilities. Such women have more to gain in comfort, muscle strength, and cardiovascular fitness than others do. Consultation with an interested and knowledgeable physiatrist or physical therapist is needed, but the physician's encouragement is essential.

Equipment and Facilities. Simple equipment at home will usually be used most regularly. Of course, costs vary with the features desired. Basic equipment at home is often less expensive than health club memberships, although some women need the stimulus of group activity. Enjoyment at home can be increased by music or television, and certainly sharing this activity with a friend, spouse or grandchild is a great stimulus.

Physicians should have a simple list available of stores, equipment, and basic costs in their area. The program at the local Ys, senior citizens groups, community services and health clubs for your patients' information is most helpful.

Guidelines for Beginners

- Choose an exercise you will enjoy.
- Find a cheerful place to do it.
- Make a regular time.
- Set a goal.
- Start slowly.
- Do warm-up and slow-down exercises.
- Use a mat or rug when appropriate.
- If pain or discomfort develops, reduce levels or check with your doctor.
- Keep a record of goal, weight, time, responses.

Figure 2. Back Exercise Regimen for Osteoporosis Patients. The following exercises should be performed 5 times a week on a firm bed or padded rug. Following *each* movement, relax, lying flat with legs in starting position. Initially each exercise should be repeated once, slowly increasing to 5–10 repeats, depending on general capacity and physician recommendations. As limberness increases, the exercises can be supplemented with 50–100 partial sit-ups which should be worked up to slowly.

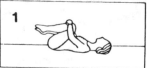

1. Lie on back with legs bent and bring both knees as close to chest as possible; hold for 5 counts.

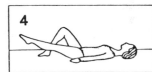

2. Bring one knee to chest while fully extending opposite leg. Hold for 5 counts.

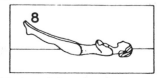

3. Bend knees and keep feet flat; press small of back against surface by tensing buttocks and stomach muscles. Hold for 5 counts.

4. With one leg bent, raise straight leg 6-12 inches off surface, keeping knee straight. Lower leg as slowly as possible.

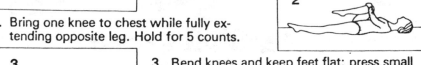

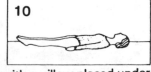

5. Bend knees and place arms across chest; raise head and shoulders. Hold for 3 counts.

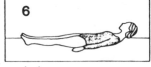

6. Extend legs with arms flat at sides; raise head and shoulders. Hold for 3 counts.

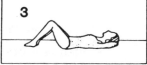

7. Extend both legs and place arms across chest; bring both legs to chest simultaneously. Return to extended position with ankles off surface.

8. Extend legs and place arms across chest; raise legs 6-12 inches. Hold for 3 counts, then lower legs slowly.

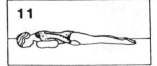

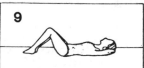

9. Place hands behind neck keeping knees bent; press elbows down to surface. Hold for 5 counts.

10. Lie on back; squeeze shoulder blades together keeping chin tucked to chest. Hold for 5 counts.

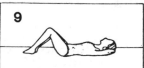

11. Lie on stomach with a pillow placed under chest; squeeze shoulder blades together, keeping chin tucked to chest. Hold for 5 counts.

Figure 3. Exercises for Low Back Pain

1

Don't overdo exercising, especially in the beginning. Start by trying the movements slowly and carefully. Don't be alarmed if the exercises cause some mild discomfort which lasts a few minutes. But if pain is more than mild and lasts more than 15 or 20 minutes, *stop* and do no further exercises until you see your doctor.

Do the exercises on a hard surface covered with a thin mat or heavy blanket. Put a pillow under your neck if it makes you more comfortable. Always start your exercises slowly—and in the order marked—to allow muscles to loosen up gradually. Heat treatments just before you start can help relax tight muscles. Follow the instructions carefully; it will be well worth the effort.

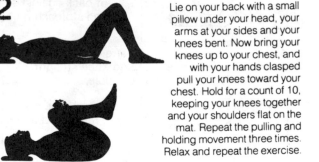

Lie on your back with your arms above your head and your knees bent. Now move one knee as far as you can toward your chest and at the same time straighten out the other leg. Go back to the original position with both knees bent, and repeat the movements, switching legs. Relax and repeat the exercise.

2

Lie on your back with a small pillow under your head, your arms at your sides and your knees bent. Now bring your knees up to your chest, and with your hands clasped pull your knees toward your chest. Hold for a count of 10, keeping your knees together and your shoulders flat on the mat. Repeat the pulling and holding movement three times. Relax and repeat the exercise.

3

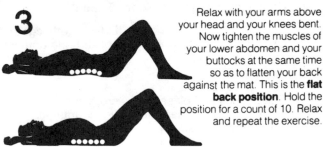

Relax with your arms above your head and your knees bent. Now tighten the muscles of your lower abdomen and your buttocks at the same time so as to flatten your back against the mat. This is the **flat back position**. Hold the position for a count of 10. Relax and repeat the exercise.

4

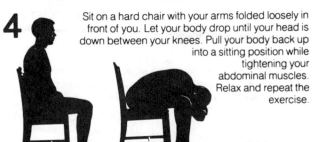

Sit on a hard chair with your arms folded loosely in front of you. Let your body drop until your head is down between your knees. Pull your body back up into a sitting position while tightening your abdominal muscles. Relax and repeat the exercise.

- Share exercising with a friend.
- Don't be discouraged.

Motivation

Motivation and continuing interest by the physician are essential to success. One should obtain a complete history and perform a physical examination before starting the patient off. Order stress testing if needed and then recommend a suitable exercise program. Emphasize to the patient the reasons for the program chosen and explain the physiologic and psychologic benefits to her. Encourage a lifetime commitment to good nutrition and exercise as preventive medicine for good health in later years. Maintain an active interest at follow-up visits (recording discussions and goals as a later reminder might be a good idea.) Positive motivation is essential. And be prepared to discuss your own personal fitness program, with your patient, because she is likely to ask!

Summary

The "aging of America" is making the postmenopausal woman an increasing part of gynecological practice. It is essential that physicians meet the needs of these older women to help them be well and active. In return, many of these older patients will remain more alert, happy and independent. Advancing age requires more attention to nutrition as caloric needs reduce, so a nutritional assessment should be a regular component of medical care in the aging. Medications which affect nutrition must be reviewed. Good oral hygiene is essential. Functional bowel problems should be distinguished from pathology. Since eating is also a social function, counsel the patient that meals should be shared with others and made enjoyable. Advancing age does not preclude a regular exercise program, the benefits of which are both physical and psychological. Motivation and continuing interest by the physician can foster a life commitment to the good nutrition and adequate exercise that will make the older woman healthier, happier, and independent.

Bibliography

Hickler, R.B. and Wayne, S. Nutrition and the elderly. American Family Physician 29:137–145, 1984.

Moghissi, K.S. and Evans, T.N. Nutritional Impacts on Women Throughout Life With Emphasis on Reproduction. Harper and Row, Hagerstown, MD, 1977.

Levenson, S.M. (Ed.) Nutritional Assessment—Present Status, Future Directions and Prospects. Ross Conferences on Medical Research, 1981, Ross Laboratories, Columbus, OH.

Notelovitz, M. and Ware, M. Stand Tall! The Informed Women's Guide to Preventing Osteoporosis. Triad Publishing Co., Gainesville, FL, 1982.

Schrier, R.W. Clinical Internal Medicine in the Aged. W.B. Saunders, Philadelphia, 1982.

Shangold, M.M. How Exercise Benefits Older Women. Contemporary Ob-Gyn 19:81–86, 1982.

3

THE ESTROGEN-DEFICIENT WOMAN

ALVIN F. GOLDFARB, M.D.

As our population slowly ages in the course of the next two decades, there will be a shift in the numbers of individuals entering middle years and beyond. In the United States today, approximately 40 million women are postmenopausal, and each of these women can look forward to a further life expectancy averaging 28 years. In spite of these facts, the implications of treatment or nontreatment for the menopausal and postmenopausal woman with sex steroid hormones have constituted the subject of only a few controlled statistically valid investigations. As we know, women are unusual among mammals in that most of them survive long beyond the end of their reproductive capabilities. With the loss of reproductive capability comes a profound change in the patient's endocrine milieu, with a marked decline in total body reproduction of estrogens.[1]

A review by Utian indicated that 75 to 85% of women ultimately have symptomatology referable to estrogen deprivation, yet only 10 to 15% of them seek medical attention for these complaints.[2] During the past two decades, some authors have been recommending that all women receive estrogen replacement therapy from the onset of the decline in their own endogenous estrogen production until their death.

Human Sexuality

Female sexual functioning during the menopausal years is extremely variable and depends on the woman's general psychic state and her relationship with her husband. The abrupt cessation of ovarian reproductive capability produces a drastic drop in the circulating levels of estrogen and progesterone. These endocrine changes are accompanied in many, but by no means all, women by the familiar irritability, depression, emotional instability, and aggressive behavior in the menopause.[3] A similar emotional crisis or period of "tension" is experienced by a small number of women during their monthly "mini-menopause."

The effect on libido of withdrawal of estrogens is, again, extremely variable. Clearly, if a woman is depressed, irritable, and insecure, she is not likely to be very interested in sex. Although some report a decrease in sexual desire, many women actually feel an increase in erotic appetite during the menopausal years. As one ages, sexual activity relates to the woman's good health and the health of her partner.

Again, the fate of libido seems to depend on a constellation of factors that characterize this period, including physiologic changes, sexual opportunity, and diminution of inhibition. From a purely physiologic standpoint, libido should theoretically increase at menopause, because the action of the woman's androgens, which is not materially affected by the menopause, is now unopposed by estrogen. Indeed, some women do seem to behave in this manner, especially if they are not depressed and can find interested and interesting partners. However, if the middle-aged husband is avoiding sex and if the insecure, depressed, and angry woman attributes this to her declining physical attractiveness, she too may avoid sexuality in order to spare herself the pain of frustration or rejection.

After the 50s, the postmenopausal years of female sexual responsiveness also show great individual variation. Women of this age group depend for their sexual expression on a dwindling supply of men whose sexual needs have declined markedly. A woman who has regular sexual opportunity tends to maintain her sexual responsiveness. Without such opportunity, sexuality declines markedly. Apart from the effect of opportunity, a slow, gradual physical decline in sexual drive seems to occur in women as well as men. Actually, age-related trophic changes of the body, and specifically the genitalia and breasts, are more profound in women than in men and are caused by postmenopausal endocrine changes. Paradoxically, these relatively severe physical changes are reflected by comparatively minimal changes in the libidinous aspects of female sexuality.

Endocrinology of the Perimenopausal Years

The most common physiologic change of the perimenopause and the menopause is the demonstration of an increase in circulating levels of FSH/LH and a decrease in the concentrations of serum estradiol. Clinically, there is an often progressive shortening of total cycle length as age advances. This reflects the fact that the number of granulosa cells surrounding follicles and the number of follicles is diminishing. Thus, as the pituitary secretes its FSH, there is no binding for these hormones at the ovarian level, and consequently an increase in circulating FSH and LH occurs. It is thought that follicles which persist until the premenopausal years are relatively resistant to gonadotropin stimulation. This immediate increase in menopausal and postmenopausal FSH will remain until the seventh or eighth decade, when FSH will slowly decrease as part of the aging process.

The effect of elevated FSH and LH in the menopause has been studied in regard to its relationship to vasomotor symptomatology. Meldrum et al. concluded after a series of experiments in humans that LH, but not FSH, showed pulsatile activity closely associated with the occurrence of symptoms and skin temperature increases during hot flashes.[4] This association suggests that factors concerned with pulsatile releases of LH may be involved in the pathophysiology of hot flashes.

The ovary continues to secrete substantial quantities of androgens, principally testosterone, after the menopause, but little or no estradiol. The serum levels of androstenedione in the menopausal woman approach the low levels found in the premenopausal woman after ovarian ablation, so there appears to be a decrease in ovarian androstenedione production, even though some secretion continues. The postmenopausal ovaries secrete higher amounts of testosterone than they do premenopausally, but the serum level of testosterone is usually unchanged, since a portion of the premenopausal woman's testosterone was formed by conversion from androstenedione, and the decrease in androstenedione leads to a reduced amount converted to testosterone. The excess in the levels of pituitary gonadotropins, which is due to the reduction of circulating estrogens, stimulates the ovarian stroma to increase its secretion of testosterone.

The circulating estrogen of most importance in postmenopausal women is estrone, which is principally derived from peripheral conversion of androstenedione with a small contribution for ovarian stromal secretion. Approximately 1.3% of circulating androstenedione is peripherally converted to estrone in premenopausal women; and the adipose tissue is implicated as the principal site in this conversion.[5] There is a positive correlation between weight and serum estrone levels, further supporting the importance of adipose tissue in this conversion.

Edman and MacDonald observed that with advancing body weight, there was an increase in the extent of conversion of androstenedione to estrone.[6] No difference was noted, however, in the extent of conversion between the ovulatory and the anovulatory groups that were matched for body weight. The conversion percentage is twice as high (2.7%) as premenopausally.

The postmenopausal ovary makes very little contribution to the levels of circulating estrogens de nova, but peripheral conversion of androstenedione to estrone accounts for most of the circulating estrogen production. Using the steroid kinetic methodology described by Siiteri and MacDonald,[7] as well as others, proof has readily been demonstrated for the increased production of estrone occurring in extraglandular aromatization, either as a result of increased extensive conversion of androstenedione to estrone or by increased production of androstenedione in women with obesity, advanced age, liver disease, polycystic ovarian disease, and ovarian stromal tumors.[7] These are pathophysiologic conditions that result in excess estrogen production. Age was a compounding factor in estrone production in the obese postmenopausal woman when compared with obese premenopausal women. It can be concluded that both advancing age and obesity are associated with increased production of estrone by means of increased aromatization.

Alterations in thyroid and adrenal function are not influenced by the climacteric. Adrenal steroid production begins to decrease with aging beyond the seventh decade in life. Thyroid hormone production is also dependent upon aging. This gland is the last of the endocrine glands to slowly lose function. There is no increase in diabetes associated with the climacteric.

Estrogen and Cancer

During the past decade, much has been written about the epidemiologic controversy involving estrogen therapy and carcinoma of the endometrium. Numerous authors, using retrospective data and case-reported studies, have suggested a possible causal relationship between estrogen increase—both exogenous and endogenous—and endometrial carcinoma.[8-11]

However, Horwitz and Feinstein, on epidemiologic and statistical grounds, decried the method for case control studies of estrogen users and the relationship to the incidence of endometrial carcinoma.[12]

Recently, Gambrell et al. reviewed four years' experience with a progestogen challenge test designed to identify women at the greatest risk for endometrial cancer.[13] In this test, patients were given either 5 mg Norlutate or 10 mg Provera for ten consecutive days each month. The progestogen was continued for as long as withdrawal bleeding was present. The use of the progestogen challenge test, according to these authors, can reduce the risk for endometrial cancer in both estrogen-treated postmenopausal women and women with increased amounts of endogenous estrogen premenopausally. This is exemplified by treating endometrial hyperplasia with progestogens and thereby preventing its progression to invasive endometrial carcinoma. To achieve this result, at least ten days of progestogen therapy are necessary each month.

MacDonald et al. identified all cases of endometrial carcinoma in Olmsted County, Minnesota, for a 30-year period from 1945 through 1974.[14] In this series, 145 patients with endometrial carcinoma were matched with 680 controls. The estimated relative risk of endometrial cancer associated with conjugated estrogen treatment given for six months or longer, was 4.9, and this increased to 7.9 with exposure for three years or longer. When a daily dose of conjugated estrogens was 1.25 mg or more and the administration was continuous, the risk was further increased. An estrogen-free period of only two years returns the relative risk for endometrial cancer to the level of risk for nonusers. Fortunately, the estrogen-cancer link seems to hold only for well-differentiated, clinically early lesions. The prevalence of stage I, AG I lesions is either a tribute to good medical surveillance of these patients or a reflection of the fact that estrogen-promoted tumors are of inherently low virulence. There appears to be no relationship between estrogens and genital cancers other than endometrial carcinoma.

Estrogens have also been suggested as a risk factor for the development of breast cancer. Recent studies by Hulka do not support any increase in the risk of breast cancer associated with estrogen use.[15] This observation can be supported further by Bland and associates, who could find no shift toward malignant disease in mammographic parenchymal patterns after long-term estrogen therapy.[16] There are no epidemiologic data at present which demonstrate a strong correlation between estrogen use and malignant disease of the breast.

Estrogens and Osteoporosis

A number of well-controlled studies have shown conclusively that estrogen-deficient states lead directly to bone loss and that, surprisingly, small doses of estrogen prevent this loss.[17-19] In one recent study, a long-acting progestogen is reported to have similar protective value.[20] Unlike other diseases associated with osteoporosis, *postmenopausal osteoporosis is a preventable public health problem*. Although black women are not susceptible to this condition (no one knows why), millions of white, yellow, and brown-skinned women are affected each year. These women suffer fractures of the vertebrae, wrists, and hips. They often have chronic pain, invalidism, deformity, and loss of height, and many thousands of them die each year or are permanently incapacitated by preventable hip fractures.

Osteoporosis is defined as insufficient bone mass. This reduction in bone mass is seen characteristically in three conditions: 1) the menopause of post-oophorectomy, 2) Cushing's syndrome, and 3) immobilization. However, these three types of osteoporosis are very different from each other clinically, genetically, and even radiologically, affecting different bones to differing degrees and actually constituting three separate diseases.

Age-related bone loss occurs in both sexes, but it begins much earlier and the rate of loss is much greater in women. The end result is that women who have smaller, lighter skeletons than men on the average, have already lost half of their bone mass by age 70, when most men are just beginning to show their first significant evidence of bone loss.

The most common of the symptomatic osteoporoses is the postmenopausal type. It is not known precisely how many millions of women are affected. What is certain is that throughout the world, elderly women can be observed bent over and walking slowly with great difficulty, obviously in pain. Radiologic examination of such women shows vertebral compressions, kyphosis, mobilization of spongiosa, and generalized thinning of the cortices. Collapsed vertebrae and kyphosis explain why so many women lose height as they age.

The fragility of the female skeleton, as evidenced by fractures of the vertebrae, wrists, and hips after age 50, was reported almost a century and a half ago. It was validated in 1962 by Alfram and Bauer.[21] In Scandinavian women, the frequency of hip fracture after age 65 doubles every five years, attaining the astonishingly high figure of 40% after age 80. In this country, data from three separate sources agree that 120,000 to 150,000 hip fractures in white American women occur every year resulting in 15,000 deaths—so that hip fracture ranks as the twelfth leading cause of death in the United States.[22,23]

The mechanism of action in the development of postmenopausal osteoporosis is estrogen-dependent and is not related to calcium and phosphorus metabolism. Estrogens do not increase the rate of bone formation, but reduce the rate of bone destruction. In a recent study, Heaney and co-workers have shown that restraint of bone resorption is lost promptly at the menopause, so that the average untreated woman at the menopause shows a 20% increase in the rate of bone resorption.[24] They also found that 18.8 mg ethylestradiol or its equivalent taken daily suffices to prevent this menopausal bone loss.

In long-term studies of postmenopausal women with advanced pathologic osteoporosis, Gordon and Vaughn advocate full replacement doses of estrogen (1.25 mg conjugated estrogen or its equivalent for 20 to 25 consecutive days each month) to prevent bone resorption.[25] When they were placed on this program, these women were soon able to resume normal or near-normal physical activity, although many had gone through an extended period of relative immobilization and invalidism. In addition, the rate of fracturing was slowed considerably. Gordon further points out that since estrogens are not anabolic for the human female skeleton, the amount of bone mass that can be restored is limited, so it is preferable to begin treatment before an excessive amount of bone tissue has been lost. The authors rather strongly suggest that before estrogen replacement is started, it is important that the patient and the physician agree that this is a lifelong commitment. When patients are taken off estrogen therapy, the progression of the disease recurs. Bone formation rate requires a considerable time to return to pretreatment level. Bone resorption rate appears to increase immediately after estrogen is stopped. All the gains of estrogen treatment will probably be lost within a relatively short time after the hormone has been withdrawn.

Hutchinson et al. conducted a case-controlled study in a

population of 2,609 women aged 40 or older, admitted to an orthopedic service during a 3-year period, in order to evaluate whether postmenopausal estrogen use protects against fractures of the hip and distal radius.[26] Analysis of the data on estrogen use in 157 matched case-controlled pairs gave an odds ratio for protection of 1.5 if the individual had taken at least 0.3 mg or an unknown dose of conjugated estrogen for 6 months or longer, starting after the menopause. If "exposure" was defined as starting estrogens within 5 years of the menopause, the ratio rose to 2.6. Estrogen use, as ascertained from interviews of 80 case-controlled pairs, increased the ratio to as high as 3.8 for exposure starting within 5 years of the menopause. A blind review of lateral x-ray films of the chest showed the prevalence of osteoporosis in fracture cases to be 32% and in controlled cases only 15%. These findings constitute epidemiologic evidence for the view that exogenous estrogens protect against postmenopausal osteoporosis.

The site of action for estrogens in preventing osteoporosis is not completely clear. There is a growing body of data suggesting that the fundamental cause of postmenopausal osteoporosis is loss of estrogenic restraining on collagenolysis. Estrogen receptors have not been found in bone, and several studies have shown that estrogens and androgens failed to restrain bone resorption in vitro. Conversely, in vitro administration of estrogen reduced collagenolysis in bones placed in tissue culture. Klotz and co-workers suggest that this paradox would be solved if estrogens were shown to exert an indirect effect on bone by increasing the production of calcitonin since calcitonin is known to inhibit bone resorption in vitro.[27]

The diagnosis of postmenopausal osteoporosis is dependent on methods used for measuring bone mass: for example, cortical thickness, photon absorptiometry, radiographic densitometry, CAT scan. The differential diagnosis of pathologic osteoporosis can sometimes present great difficulties. The most common conditions confused with postmenopausal osteoporosis, because of a similar roentgen appearance, are metastatic cancer and myeloma. These can often, but not always, be differentiated by appropriate clinical and laboratory examination. Uncomplicated osteoporosis does not alter the circulating levels of serum alkaline phosphatase, calcium, or the electrophoretic protein pattern. Anemia is not associated with uncomplicated osteoporosis.

An association of osteoporosis with slender body habitus has been suggested as playing a role in the more frequent development of osteoporosis in slender postmenopausal women. In a recent study by Frumar and co-workers, circulating estrogen levels were shown to correlate with percent ideal weight in postmenopausal women, and both estradiol and estrone levels correlated positively with an index of obesity.[28] Estrogen levels were not significantly related to age, time since menopause, or height. Slender body habitus was associated with lower circulating estrogen levels. Using a urinary calcium-creatinine ratio as an index of bone resorption, there was a negative correlation with body weight, which in turn correlated positively with serum estrogen levels. It can be concluded that overweight women are protected from osteoporosis by virtue of their higher estrogen levels as a result of peripheral aromatization of androgens in adipose tissue. Therapeutically, it might be concluded that slender women might be especially appropriate candidates for estrogen replacement. This added information can now be placed in proper perspective in terms of the management of osteoporosis in the postmenopausal female.

The development of osteoporosis probably involves many factors, including hormonal, nutritional, physical, and perhaps other unknown effects. Although the influences of hormones alone on bone are varied and complex, a dominant effect is the apparently indirect action of estrogens in suppressing bone resorption—an action that is reduced after the menopause. The rate of bone loss is approximately 0.5% per year after the age of 40; in the postmenopausal woman, the rate accelerates to 1% or more per year—a rate that continues for about 5 years.[29]

Factors other than estrogen influence the development of osteoporosis. Among these factors are nutrition, more specifically calcium metabolites. Calcium absorption decreases with age and is lower in osteoporotic patients than in normal subjects of the same age. Elderly patients and those with osteoporosis have required higher amounts of dietary calcium to prevent a negative calcium balance. Since calcium concentrations in serum and body fluid must be maintained for normal neuromuscular function, as well as other functions, exogenous calcium deficiency must be compensated for from skeletal reserves.[30]

Osteoporosis is an example of a disease that may be preventable in many women if physicians and the public become better informed. Any woman approaching or passing through the menopause is susceptible. The management of the problem may well relate to both hormonal and nutritional supplementation, and in addition, frequent weight-bearing exercise, such as walking, should complement the first two approaches in suppressing bone resorption and may stimulate bone formation.

Management of Estrogen Replacement Therapy

Before instituting estrogen replacement therapy, a review of the risks versus the benefits should be individualized for each patient placed in a treatment program. The risks of estrogen replacement therapy can be related to an increased risk factor of endometrial carcinoma, the development of gallbladder disease, and a possible increase in cardiovascular disease or breast cancer. The benefits relate to the prevention or control of coronary artery disease, vasomotor symptoms, insomnia, atrophic changes of the lower reproductive tract, and osteoporosis.

Before instituting any estrogen replacement therapy program, the patient should provide a complete history and undergo a physical examination including Pap smear and laboratory studies as indicated. In addition, individuals who exhibit signs of hirsutism, obesity, diabetes, or hypertension may need a more detailed evaluation and careful follow-up before being placed on estrogen therapy. The risks versus benefits of therapy should be reviewed with each individual.

In the menopausal woman who has abnormal uterine bleeding, that is, uterine bleeding that is unpredictable, prolonged or excessive, histologic evaluation of the endometrium prior to instituting estrogen replacement is mandatory. In addition, in any individual who develops abnormal bleeding while receiving estrogen replacement therapy, an endometrial evaluation prior to the resumption of any steroid treatment program is essential.

All patients receiving estrogen replacement should be seen regularly, usually at 6- to 12-month intervals. At these examinations, blood pressure should be taken, a breast and pelvic examination performed, and an evaluation of the effectiveness of treatment noted. With this information, the effective minimum dose of estrogen replacement can be established. Papanicolaou smears should be taken annually; any abnormality in bleeding necessitates a commitment to the evaluation of this symptom.

It is recommended that estrogen replacement therapy, and all treatment programs, be given in cyclic fashion. Cyclic estrogen therapy should be interrupted at least every other cycle with sequential progesterone therapy. Generally, oral preparations are preferred to those given by injection or implantation. Parenteral estrogens should rarely be used. The lowest effective estrogen dose for the patient as her own control should be utilized. Most patients require between 0.625 mg to 1.25 mg of conjugated estrone sulfate, or its equivalent, per day for adequate replacement.

Estrogen is taken 21 to 25 days in each cycle; sequential Medoxy progesterone should be added for the last seven days of each cycle. The dose of the progesterone is 5 to 10 mg a day. Using this regimen, the patient is not at increased risk for the development of endometrial carcinoma.[30]

If intermenstrual spotting, staining, or unusual bleeding develops, sampling of the endometrium is mandatory. Estrogen therapy should be stopped until the histologic evaluation of the tissue is completed. The patient may restart cyclic estrogen-progesterone therapy after a 4-week hiatus, should the histology be normal.

The patient being treated for vasomotor instability should be re-evaluated 12 to 18 months after starting treatment. At that point the physician must decide whether to continue treating this patient with substitutional therapy.

Prophylaxis and treatment of osteoporosis with estrogen is in state of flux at the present moment. There are individuals who believe that all menopausal and postmenopausal women should be maintained on cyclic doses of estrogen, as low as 0.3 mg daily, from the first to the twenty-fifth day of every month for the remainder of their lives. There are not enough data as yet to support this concept.

The use of estrogen therapy in managing atrophic vaginitis and urethritis is usually mandatory to prevent symptoms and to improve the quality of life. Employing vaginal estrogen creams to control this problem is usually a first line of defense. Estrogens are absorbed by the vagina and may cause irregular bleeding. I usually reserve this form of treatment for the very elderly who have asymptomatic vaginitis and/or urethritis; otherwise, I prefer cyclic estrogen and progesterone.

Some women for whom substitutional estrogen replacement is contraindicated have severe menopausal symptoms. These patients can be helped, on occasion, with sedatives, psychopharmacologic agents, progestins, and rarely, androgens. The daytime sedative that is most commonly used is one combining phenobarbital and belladonna. Psychopharmacologic agents, as a rule, are of minimum value in treating symptoms related to an estrogen-deficient state.

Androgen therapy has been described as being of value for the markedly asthenic anoretic type of menopausal patient with symptoms, who may also require anabolic steroids. Androgens have also been described as increasing libido. Androgen therapy may produce side-effects, such as acne, hirsutism, and more seriously, irreversible clitoromegaly.

In the patient who has been treated for endometrial or breast cancer and in whom estrogens are contraindicated, progestational compounds may be of value. The progestins that should be used are those that are related biochemically to the pregnane series (C-21 progestins). These compounds, in proper dosage, relieve the vasomotor symptoms. There is no doubt that large doses of progestins control vasomotor instability, but they have no effect on bone resorption or on causing growth in the atrophic vagina.

Philosophically, the woman who is menopausal and post-menopausal requires an empathetic physician to listen well, evaluate well, and make an educated judgment about therapeutics. As we learn more about the middle years and aging, there will be changes in philosophy regarding therapeutic programs. The most important thing that can be said is that we are just beginning to understand the role of estrogens as treatment in the postmenopausal woman on a long-term basis. As yet, there have been no reports that would contraindicate using small amounts of estrogen continuously to minimize osteoporosis and thus prevent the serious problem of hip fracture and its sequelae. The individual who has an atrophic vagina and urethra and is symptomatic certainly requires estrogen supplementation on a regular basis. When the individual is given estrogens in sequential fashion, with intermittent progesterone therapy, the risk factor for endometrial carcinoma is no greater than in the individual who has never been given substitutional estrogens.

REFERENCES

1. Ryan KS, Gibson DD. Menopause and Aging. DHEW Publication No. (NIH) 73:319, 1972.
2. Utian WH. Current status of menopause and postmenopausal therapy—help or hazard. N Engl J Med *301*:464, 1979.
3. Gerder LC, Sonnendecker EW, Polakow ES. Psychological changes effected by estrogen-progesten and clomidine treatment in climacteric women. Am J Obstet Gynecol *142*:192, 1982.
4. Meldrum DR, Erpik Y, Lu JKM, Jude HL. Objectively recorded hot flushes in patients with pituitary insufficiency, Clin Endocrinol Metab *52*:684–687, 1981.
5. Speroff L, Judd HL, Richart RM, Ziel HK. Symposium: The estrogen replacement controversy. Contemp Obstet Gynecol *8*:143, 1976.
6. Edman CD, MacDonald PC. Effect of obesity on conversion of plasma androstenedione to estrone in ovulatory and anovulatory young women. Am J Obstet Gynecol *130*:456, 1978.
7. Siiteri PK, MacDonald PC. Role of extraglandular estrogen in human endocrinology. In *Handbook of Physiology*. Sec. 7, Endocrinology. Vol. 2, Pt. I. Edited by R. Greep and EB Astwood. Washington, D.C., American Physiological Society, 1973.
8. Ziel HK, Finkle WD. Increased risk of endometrial carcinoma among users of conjugated estrogens. N Engl J Med *293*:1167, 1976.
9. Weiss NS, Szekely DR, Austin DF. Increasing Incidence of endometrial carcinoma in the United States. N Engl J Med *294*:1259, 1976.
10. Mack TM, Pike MC, Henderson BE et al. Estrogens and endometrial cancer in a retirement community. N Engl J Med *294*:1262, 1976.
11. McDonald TW, Annegers JF, O'Fallon WM et al. Exogenous estrogen and endometrial carcinoma: case-control and incidence study. Am J Obstet Gynecol *127*:572, 1977.
12. Horwitz RE, Feinstein AR. Alternate analytic methods for case-control studies of estrogens and endometrial cancer. N Engl J Med *299*:1089, 1978.
13. Gambrell RD, Massey FM, Castareda TA, Ugenas AJ, Ricci CA, Wright JM. Use of progestogen challenge test to reduce risk of endometrial cancer. Obstet Gynecol *55*:732–738, 1980.
14. McDonald TW, Annegers JF, O'Fallon MW et al. Exogenous estrogen and endometrial carcinoma: case-control and incidence study. Am J Obstet Gynecol *127*:572, 1977.
15. Hulka BS. Effect of exogenous estrogen on postmenopausal women: the epidemiologic evidence. Obstet Gynecol *35*:389:198.
16. Bland KI, Buchannan JB, Weissberg BG. The effects of exogenous estrogen replacement therapy of the breast: breast cancer risk and mammographic parenchymal patterns. Cancer *45*:3027, 1980.
17. Gordan GS, Vaughan C. Clinical Management of the Osteoporoses. Acton, Mass, Publishing Sciences Group, 1976.
18. Gordon GS. Drug treatment of the osteoporoses. Ann Rev Pharmacol Toxicol *18*:253, 1978.

19. Meema S, Bunker ML, Meema H. Preventive effect of estrogen on post-menopausal bone loss. Arch Intern Med *135*:1436, 1975.
20. Lindsay R, Hart DM, et al. Comparative effects of estrogen and progestogen on bone loss in postmenopausal women. Clin Sci *54*:193, 1978.
21. Alfram PA, Bauer CH. Epidemiology of fractures of the forearm. J Bone Joint Surg *44-A*:105–114, 1962.
22. Gallagher JC, Melton LJ et al. Epidemiology of fractures of the proximal femur in Rochester, Minnesota. Clin Orthop, 1980.
23. National Center for Health Statistics: Inpatient utilization of short-stay hospitals by diagnosis, United States, 1975. Vital and Health Statistics Series 13, No. 35. DHEW Pub. No. (PHS) 78-1786. Washington, D.C., US Government Printing Office, April, 1978.
24. Heaney RP, Recker RR, Saville PD. Menopausal changes in bone remodeling. J Lab Clin Med *92*:964, 1978.
25. Gordon GS, Vaughn C. Sex steroids in the clinical management of osteoporosis. In Clinical Use of Sex Steroids (Edited by James R. Givens). Yearbook Publishers, 1980, pp 69–94.
26. Hutchinson JA, Polansky SM, Feinstein AR. Postmenopausal estrogens protect against fractures of hip and distal radius. Lancet 2:705–709, 1979.
27. Klotz HP, Delorme ML, et al. Hormones sexuelles et secretion de calcitonine. Sem Hop *51*:1333, 1975.
28. Frumar AM, Meldrum DR, Geola F, Shamanki IM, Tataryn IV, Deftos LJ, Judd HL. Relationship of fasting urinary calcium to circulating estrogens and body weight in postmenopausal women. J Clin Endocrinol Metab *40*:70–75, 1980.
29. Amin DM, Khaire MRA, Norton J, Johnston CC, Jr. Age and activity effects on rate of bone mineral loss. J Clin Meth *58*:716–21, 1976.
30. Hammond CB, Jelovsik FR, Lee KL et al. Effects of long-term estrogen replacement therapy: II Neoplasia. Am J Obstet Gynecol *133*:537, 1979.

4

CARCINOMA OF THE BREAST

C. PAUL HODGKINSON, M.D.

"Geriatrics is that branch of medicine which treats all problems peculiar to old age and aging, including the clinical problems of senescence and senility" (Dorland's Medical Dictionary).

By definition, carcinoma of the breast is not a geriatric problem per se because it is a disease not peculiar to old age. However, its presence does complicate the management of patients with geriatric problems. There are questions to be asked: Is there a consensus regarding the age when geriatric problems begin? Does the process of aging alter the behavior of breast cancer, and if so, does this alter treatment?

It has been calculated that 1 out of every 13 patients (7%) who walk into the office of the obstetrician-gynecologist will, at some time in her life, develop carcinoma of the breast. Presumably this calculation was based on the average life span of the human female, which in 1980 was calculated to reach 72 years. But many women live many years longer. It has also been calculated that a woman who achieves the age of 72 years has an average life expectancy of an additional 12.6 years;[1] at 80, the added life expectancy is 8.2 years (Table 4-1). The elderly represent an increasing percentage of the population; an estimated 11% are over 65 years of age.

TABLE 1.   LIFE EXPECTANCY OF THE AMERICAN FEMALE

Age (yr)	Life Expectancy (yr)	Age (yr)	Life Expectancy (yr)
70	13.9	78	9.2
71	13.3	79	8.7
72	12.6	80	8.2
73	12.0	81	7.8
74	11.4	82	7.3
75	10.8	83	6.9
76	10.3	84	6.5
77	9.7	85	6.1

From the National Center for Health, Rockville, Md.

For this project, elderly has arbitrarily been defined as those women approaching the average age of life expectancy: 70 to 72 years. Consideration has also been given to patients who developed carcinoma of the breast after the age of 70 years. They were divided into two groups: the *"young" geriatric patient*, ranging in age from 70 to 80, and the *"old" geriatric patient*, from 80 years on. However, some patients at 80 are in considerably better health than some at 75. Approximately 75% of females who die at age 75 die of heart disease and stroke, while only 15% die of cancer.[1]

The report derives from an ongoing study of breast cancer since 1946 involving 255 patients. It is a personal report, because all of these patients were operated on and followed by me. Only 3 patients have been lost to follow-up.

Age Incidence

The age range for carcinoma of the breast in the present series was from 30 to 89 years, with a mean of 55 years. As shown in Figure 4-1, 35 or 14% of the cancers occurred in patients aged 70 years or older. Of the 35 elderly patients, 25 (74%) were less than 80 years old and were classified as "young" geriatric patients. All of the patients under 80 were apparently in good mental and physical health. They performed their own work, did their own shopping, and moved freely in society, even driving their automobiles. They were considered suitable for radical or modified radical breast surgery.

Ten (26%) were 80 years or older and were classified as "old" geriatric patients (Figure 4-1). All of the patients in this group had some limiting physical or mental disability which increased the risk for anesthesia and extensive surgery. Many of these patients had diabetes, or a history of previous heart attacks, stroke, severe arteriosclerotic cardiovascular disease, or disabling arthritis.

Surgery in the Aged

Surgery in the patient over 70 years of age must be given serious contemplation. Although surgery of the breast does not involve entering the body cavities unless resection of the internal mammary lymph nodes is performed, it is a formidable operation for the geriatric patient. A complete medical survey should be taken preoperatively, with particular atten-

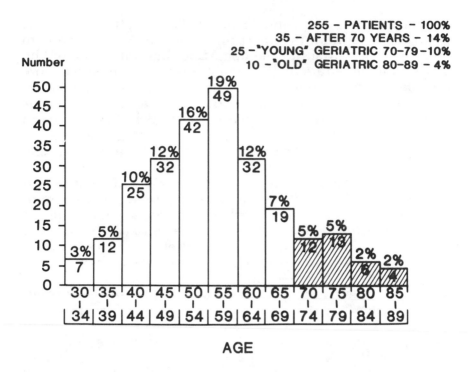

255 – PATIENTS – 100%
35 – AFTER 70 YEARS – 14%
25 – "YOUNG" GERIATRIC 70-79 – 10%
10 – "OLD" GERIATRIC 80-89 – 4%

Figure 4-1. Age incidence of carcinoma of the breast.

tion to cardiovascular problems. Many patients in this group are on various drug regimens, particularly antihypertensive medication. Observing the electrolyte balance is very important, especially for low potassium levels. Insulin doses must be carefully regulated for those who are diabetic. Postoperative sedation must be administered with great care: only the smallest doses should be given because what is an average dose for a younger patient may cause severe mental confusion in the elderly. In these cases, protective nursing care is imperative. In unfamiliar surroundings, confused elderly patients may fall while attempting to go to the bathroom or get "lost" and wander from their rooms. Early ambulation is of course essential to minimize thromboembolic problems.

All surgical procedures should be performed in a meticulous manner, but this is especially true for the geriatric patient. The greatest care must be taken to provide complete hemostasis both during and following surgery. Because most of these patients have severe arteriosclerosis, small arterioles fail to contract and tend to bleed more profusely than in younger patients. It is important to remember the old adage, "The elderly will stand the operation, but not the complications." Postoperatively, care must be taken to observe blood chemistry, intake and output, and electrolyte values, since geriatric patients tend to have more drainage of serum after breast surgery than do younger patients. Selecting the operative procedure for the breast cancer patient ought to be determined by the physical status of the patient, the expected longevity according to age, and the stage of the cancer.

Most geriatric patients, if in reasonably good health, will tolerate modified radical mastectomy. In the series under discussion, radical or modified radical mastectomy was performed 21 times. All of the patients eventually healed well with minimal complications. Four developed arm edema, for which a Jobst compression sleeve was required. There were no operative deaths. Based on this study and the reports of others, modified radical mastectomy is the operation of choice for geriatric patients. Lymph node metastasis occurs in this age group with almost the same frequency as it does in younger patients. Kessler and Seton[1] reported lymph node metastasis in 24% of Columbia A lesions[2] and 68% of Columbia B lesions in patients over age 70. The incidence reported by Haagensen et al.[3] was 32% for Columbia Group A and 76% for Group B. In our series of 35 patients, pathologic specimens from 32 were available for axillary lymph node determination; metastasis was noted in only 19%.

For some geriatric patients with breast cancer, simple mastectomy with high dissection of the accessible axillary fat, with or without postoperative radiation therapy, may be the procedure of choice. In 4 of 14 patients who underwent this procedure, this decision was based on the advanced stage of the cancer. In each instance the cancer involved the entire breast (Stage T-4), and operation was performed to avoid breast ulceration. Three of these patients have died of their carcinoma. One is living after undergoing radiation therapy; her cancer involved the entire breast, and a CAT scan showed that the tumor had penetrated the chest wall but not the pleura. She had observed her breast lump for over 3 years, but had delayed treatment because she thought her death would occur from some cause other than her cancer of the breast. When this did not happen and she began to have pain and skin changes, she sought medical treatment. She has survived one year without evidence of systemic metastasis. Selection of simple mastectomy for the remaining 10 patients was based on impaired physical status in 4 and advanced age (over 80 years) in 6. After the age of 80, life expectancy is reduced to 8 years, and in patients with T 1-2 N-O the likelihood of dying from heart disease or stroke is considerably greater than the likelihood of dying from cancer. All of these 10 patients are living without evidence of metastasis. The oldest patient is 91, and all but 2 are in their 80s.

Staging

Although there are various methods of staging breast cancer, the technique used for this series was the TNM system adopted by the Joint Committee for Cancer Staging.[4] All patients subjected to modified radical or radical mastectomy and those subjected to simple mastectomy with high dissection of the axillary fat were staged postoperatively as follows:

Tumor Size
TIS—Lobular carcinoma in situ
T-0—No palpable tumor
T-1—2 cm or less
T-2—2-4 cm
T-3—4-7 cm
T-4—over 7 cm

Lymph Node Involvement
N-0 —None
N-1 —Less than 10% involved
N-2 —10 to 50% involved
N-3 —More than 50% but less than 100% involved
N-4 —100% involved
N-X—Not staged (simple mastectomy)

One tumor was staged TIS. One tumor, not clinically palpable, was detected by mammography and was staged T-0. The remaining were all palpable and were staged as follows

T-1 N-0 —12
T-2 N-1 — 3
T-1 N-3 — 1
T-3 N-X— 1

```
 T-2  N-0 —  6
 T-2  N-2 —  2
 T-2  N-4 —  1
 T-2  N-X—  3
 T-3  N-1 —  1
 T-3  N-X—  1
 T-4  N-4 —  1
 T-4  N-X—  1
```

TOTAL 33

Results of Treatment

One patient has been lost to follow-up. Five patients (14%) have died of cancer and 5 (14%) of diseases unrelated to cancer. Of those who died of cancer, 3 had extensive metastasis to the regional lymph nodes at the time of their initial operation. Two cases, after simple mastectomy for huge T-3-4 tumors, were staged T-3-4 N-X. No patient with negative axillary metastasis has died of cancer. Of the 6 patients with known axillary metastasis, 2 patients, one aged 71 and staged T-3 N-1 and the other aged 73 and staged T-2 N-2, are living without evidence of recurrence after 4 and 3 years, respectively. Both were subjected to modified radical mastectomy followed by radiation therapy. The cancer-free survival rate of this series was 86%. This compares favorably with the report from Columbia Hospital by Kessler and Seton,[1] who reported 82% survival in 71 patients over the age of 70 years. Herbsman et al.[5] reported cancer-free survival in 86% of those with localized disease.

Attitude of Geriatric Patient toward Breast Cancer

It is apparent from this study that many elderly patients become complacent toward breast cancer. Although 12 (34%) of the tumors observed were less than 2 cm in diameter, 21 patients, when first observed, had tumors considerably larger. Five (15%) neglected to seek medical care until almost the entire breast was involved. Except for 2 tumors that were not clinically palpable, all of the others were palpable and many were known to the patient. One patient had known of the tumor for 3 years! Except for 5, the other 14 reported promptly once their tumors were discovered. Surprisingly, 14 (42%) of the tumors were first discovered on routine yearly clinical examination. In 4 of the patients who had had a previous breast cancer, the tumor in the opposite breast was discovered during routine follow-up examination. Some of the patients, when questioned, admitted doing self-examination of the breasts, but most did not practice this procedure. Usually they stated that they did not like to feel their breasts and were indecisive when they did.

This study strongly emphasizes the need for routine gynecologic examinations in older patients. I have found the "towel trick" of great value in detecting tumors that are difficult to feel. This procedure consists of stretching a freshly ironed towel over the breast and quickly sweeping the hand over the towel in all directions. By this technique areas of breast thickening appear to be accentuated. The principle of the "towel trick" is probably the same as examining the breasts with soaped hands, as advocated by Abramson.[6] Mammograms should be included in the routine yearly gynecologic examination for the elderly female as advocated by the ACS for all patients over 50. Personal experience with mammograms until about 1975 was rather discouraging because of a high percentage (54%) of false-negative reports in patients with palpable three-dimensional tumors proven to be invasive cancer. However, the results have improved in the past few years, and nonpalpable tumors have been detected by mammography with increasing frequency.

It is important to keep mammography in the proper perspective. It is improper to make a conclusive pathologic diagnosis from mammograms alone. Mammography is a screening technique for patients with nonpalpable breast tumors. In patients with three-dimensional breast masses, mammograms are of value in detecting nonpalpable tumors in the opposite breast; they should not be used as a guide to therapy. Although typical calcium deposits and hazy contour dimensions are suggestive of malignancy, their absence does not exclude malignancy. Negative mammograms are no excuse to delay surgical excision of a palpable three-dimensional breast tumor.

Comment

From analysis of 35 tumors observed in patients over the age of 70 years, it was apparent that cancer of the breast in elderly patients is a unique problem. Although this small group of patients does not compare to the larger series of retrospective patients reported by Herbsman et al.,[5] and by

Kessler and Seton,[1] the results are about the same. The series described in this report has the advantage of being an ongoing personal observation of 255 patients treated for breast cancer, with only 3 being lost to follow-up. There may be some advantage in considering geriatric breast cancer patients as two separate groups: "young" and "old" geriatric patients. There is some evidence that breast cancer is less aggressive after the age of 70, and particularly after 80. It is evident from this study and others[1,5] that, if neglected, regional metastases do occur. It is evident that radical or modified radical mastectomy is the treatment of choice for the "young" geriatric patient—and also for the "old" geriatric patient if her state of health permits. However, in this small series, for the patient over 80 simple mastectomy with high dissection of the axillary fat pad has produced very satisfactory results. With life expectancy reduced to about 7 years at age 80, simple mastectomy seems to be an acceptable procedure.

REFERENCES

1. Kessler HJ, Seton JZ. Treatment of operable breast cancer in the elderly female. Am J Surg 135:664, 1978.
2. Haagensen CD. Diseases of the Breast. 2nd Ed. Philadelphia, W.B. Saunders, 1971, p. 630.
3. Haagensen CD, Kennedy CS, Handley RS, Butcher HR, Culversen E, Williams IG, Kaae S. Treatment of early mammary carcinoma: a cooperative study. Ann Surg 157:157, 1963.
4. Clinical Staging System for Carcinoma of the Breast. The Executive Secretary American Joint Committee for Cancer Staging and End Results Reporting. 55 East Erie St., Chicago, IL 60611, 1973.
5. Herbsman H, Feldman J, Seldera J, Gardner B, Alfonso A. Survival following breast cancer surgery in the elderly. Am Cancer Soc 47:2358, 1981.
6. Abramson DL. A simplified technique for breast examination—palpation with soaped hands. GP 23:120, 1961.

5

THE AGING VULVA

EDUARD G. FRIEDRICH, JR., H.A.B., M.D., L.L.D. (HON.)

Untold numbers of aging women shun social activities and confine themselves to their homes for fear of the public embarrassment associated with vulvar pruritus. The itching stimulus leads to rubbing and scratching with inevitable excoriation as a consequence. Soreness and pain from the open fissures which then occur contribute to the misery. Those women who have remained sexually active develop dyspareunia and begin to avoid intercourse. With the passage of time, the introitus shrinks and a true kraurosis or decreased introital diameter results. The primary cause of this chain of events is a condition of the skin known as lichen sclerosus.

Little is known of the basic process responsible for this disease which was first described by the French dermatologist Hallopeau in 1887. A wide variety of skin sites may be affected: trunk, neck, back, and the male glans penis (balanitis xerotica obliterans). But the most frequently involved site is the vulva. All age groups are susceptible, including the very young.[4] But postmenopausal women are most often affected. Lichen sclerosus is therefore principally a disease of the aging woman.

For years, gynecologists have assumed that the vulvar skin in such individuals had undergone an estrogen-deprivation atrophy similar to that occurring in the vagina. It is true that the aging integument in general exhibits some degree of cutaneous atrophy with diminished glandular secretion during the climacteric. There is also a decrease in the turgor and elasticity of the skin and mucous membranes associated with the aging process. But it is erroneous to assume that these changes are simply related to a decrease in estrogen. The climacteric is not a unihormonal event.

Another source of past confusion lay in the ambiguous nomenclature frequently applied to the disease; there were no fewer than 18 synonyms by which lichen sclerosus was once described. It was logical, then, for the International Society for the Study of Vulvar Disease to focus its early attention on the establishment of a universal nomenclature. In 1976, that organization published a uniform terminology discarding the old connotations surrounding the term "leukoplakia" and substituting the concept of *dystrophy*, a word suggested by Jeffcoate to encompass the benign majority of vulvar white lesions.[13] Lichen sclerosus is then one form of vulvar dystrophy and is defined by strict histopathological criteria. The epidermis is thin and exhibits loss of the rete ridges and a disordered basal layer. There is a zone of homogenization beneath the epidermis with disruption of the normal collagen usually found in this location. Finally, a band of chronic inflammatory cells is frequently located in the deep dermis (*Fig. 1*). These three hallmarks of the disease allow the

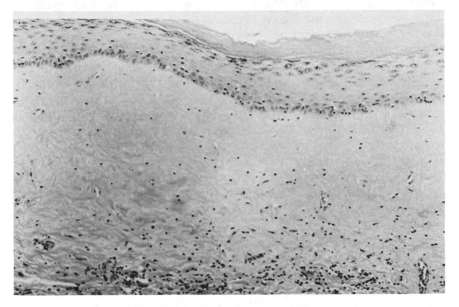

Figure 5:1. The histologic appearance of lichen sclerosus.

pathologist to classify the tissue with certainty as lichen sclerosus, so that a simple punch biopsy performed in the office under local anesthesia should be obtained from all suspect cases to confirm the diagnosis.

Clinically, lichen sclerosus causes the vulvar skin to appear pale or white. The thin glistening epidermis is easily wrinkled. Ecchymoses are frequent because of the close proximity of the fragile underlying dermal vessels to the surface. Any amount of rubbing or scratching is likely to produce this subepithelial hemorrhage. As the disease process advances, the labia minora become adherent and finally incorporated into the major vulvar folds and their independent structure is lost. The frenulum and prepuce are agglutinated and eventually bury the glans of the clitoris beneath an amorphous mass of scar-like tissue (*Fig. 2*).

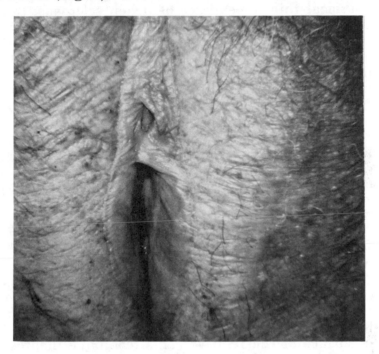

Figure 5:2. Lichen sclerosus of the vulva.

Another form of dystrophy, the hyperplastic variety, may co-exist with lichen sclerosus and constitute a so-called *mixed dystrophy*. This is an important distinction which bears on the premalignant potential of the lesion. In what has become a classic paper on the relationship of lichen sclerosus to vulvar carcinoma, Hart and his colleagues[12] noted that women with lichen sclerosus who later developed a squamous tumor did so from areas of co-existing hyperplasia. Even this is a rare event, but foci of hyperplasia should be identified and carefully followed.

For this reason, a single punch biopsy may be insufficient. The purpose of histologic sampling is twofold: to investigate the most suspicious areas and to document a representative area of change. Therefore, if the entire lesion is homogeneous in appearance, even though it may encompass a wide area, a single punch biopsy is usually adequate to represent the total change. On the other hand, if the lesion is variegated with areas of thickening, ulceration, or hyperpigmentation as well as the typical thin appearance of lichen sclerosus, further biopsies are mandatory to sample the complete disturbance.

The toluidine blue test can assist in directing the biopsies to sites of possible atypia. A vital stain, toluidine blue will become fixed to superficial nuclei present on the skin surface and will resist decolorization with acetic acid. Such nuclei are present on the surface of ulcers and also in areas of parakeratosis which may overlay foci of more significant atypia. The test is carried out by applying a 1% aqueous solution of toluidine blue-0 dye to the entire vulva. After a minute or two to allow for adequate fixation, the skin is washed gently with 1% acetic acid. Any areas of retained dye are suspect and should then be biopsied.[6] The Keyes cutaneous punch instrument 4 or 5 mm in diameter is ideally suited to this purpose. After generous infiltration with local anesthetic, using a fine needle, the instrument is applied to the skin like a cork-borer and twirled gently. The circumsected plug of tissue is then lifted with a small Adson forceps and cut free with a scissors. The tissue plug should next be placed, epidermal side upwards, on a small piece of absorbent cardboard to which it will adhere. The cardboard square is then allowed to float inverted on the surface of the fixative. This technique insures flat fixation of the skin and allows the pathologist to properly orient the section in order to obtain perpendicular tissue slices. The resultant slides allow for accurate interpretation, and confusing "tangential cuts" can be avoided.

Once a diagnosis of pure lichen sclerosus is made, the patient's fear of cancer can be put to rest. She is no more or less likely to develop vulvar carcinoma than her unaffected sister of the same age, unless the lesion is ignored and areas of hyperplasia and atypia are allowed to develop.

The management of lichen sclerosus currently rests on the empirical observation of Cinberg,[2] who noted that the condition improved with the topical application of testosterone. His work was later expanded by Williams and Richardson,[22] who in turn stimulated other investigators[7,15,19,25] to assess the efficacy of this therapy. A review of the literature now shows that 135 women out of 142 treated after biopsy improved with the use of topical testosterone. Through the years, a wide variety of treatments have been tried and discarded. None has ever approached the degree of effectiveness found with topical testosterone.

Currently, no commercial preparations of this drug are available. It must be compounded locally using testosterone propionate in sesame oil thoroughly mixed into white petrolatum at a 2 percent by weight concentration. One method of preparation requires mixing three vials of the testosterone propionate, each containing 10 cc of oil (in which is dissolved one gram of the hormone) with 120 gm of molten petrolatum. The mixture should be stirred as it cools so that separation does not occur. This amount is sufficient for about three months in most cases.

The patient is instructed to *gently* massage a small amount of the ointment into the affected skin area twice a day. On this regimen, most women will note relief of symptoms or a change in the appearance of the lesion after six months. It is very important for the patient and her physician to understand that lichen sclerosus is a slow disease process. Reversal or arrest of that process appropriately requires many months of continued medication. Once a therapeutic result has been achieved, the frequency of application may be decreased to once a day at bedtime. This dosage is continued for about a year, after which further improvement is unlikely. However, complete discontinuance of therapy results in a predictable recurrence. For this reason, continued maintenance therapy for life is recommended, using the ointment on a once-a-week basis.

The most frequent side effect to topical testosterone is clitoral hypertrophy. As the prepuce and frenulum become redefined, the enlarging glans become more prominent. By itself this is not a troublesome development. Many women, however, note a concomitant increase in libido. Again, this may pose no problem for women who remain sexually active. On the other hand, the widow of many years, whose sexuality has long been dormant, may become increasingly uncomfortable. This is especially true if she does not understand that the phenomenon is an expected result of the medication. Even with this insight, a few women are so distressed by masturbatory fantasies that they prefer to discontinue therapy. Preexisting facial hair may increase in amount and become more coarse in texture, but this is a rare side effect. At least two cases of hoarseness have also been reported, but in general, significant side effects are few and most can be managed with ease. It is important to stress that the ointment should be worked *gently* into the affected skin. Vigorous rubbing may produce hemorrhage and ulceration. In the latter event, the ointment should be discontinued and a mild cortico- steroid cream temporarily substituted until the ulcerations are completely healed.

Despite the excellent results achieved in most cases, some women fail to respond to topical testosterone. Usually this is because of inaccurate compounding of the ointment or failure in proper application. But even when these common faults are corrected, a few recalcitrant cases remain. In such instances, alternative forms of therapy should be considered.

If recurrent ulceration or severe testosterone side effects make further use of the ointment undesirable, a progesterone cream may be used instead.[14] While sometimes better tolerated, it is slower in producing therapeutic results. The cream is not commercially available and must again be compounded using 100 gm of progesterone in oil per 1 oz of Aquaphor base. Four to six ounces are generally prepared at a time and the cream is applied on a twice-a-day basis in much the same manner as the testosterone ointment.

When all topical therapy fails to produce relief from itching, alcohol injection may be offered. This technique has been successfully employed by Woodruff in 35 cases.[23] Pruritus will usually disappear after injection but the symptom of *vulvar burning is not relieved* by alcohol and, in fact, may even be aggravated. Accordingly, cases must be carefully selected. The injection technique requires some practice. If the underlying fat is inadvertently saturated with alcohol, an extensive and painful necrosis may result. Finally, some cases have had a short-lived response and the symptoms have recurred after six months to a year. Mering[17] has advocated perivulvar-perianal neurotomy procedures as a last resort for those patients who fail to respond to less drastic measures. With this technique, the major nerve supply to the vulva is surgically severed with sharp and blunt dissection, undermining the vulvar skin through two long incisions which parallel the lateral borders of the labia majora.

The lack of a simple and uniformly effective therapy stems from our ignorance of the fundamental cause of this disease. Relatively little basic research has been carried out. From tissue enzyme studies it is apparent that lichen sclerosus is not an *atrophic* process.[20] Enzymatic activity in lichen sclerotic epithelium actually exceeds that in normal postmenopausal vulvar skin. Similarly, the nuclear metabolism of the squamous epithelium is relatively active, judging from the concentration of RNA and DNA[8] and the nuclear uptake of tritiated thymidine.[24]

For many years, an immunologic defect has been thought to play a role in the development of lichen sclerosus. However, little evidence could be found to support this suspicion until Harrington[11] noted a higher incidence of tissue antibodies and auto-immune diseases in patients with lichen sclerosus than in a control population. Using direct immunofluorescence, Bushkell and his colleagues[1] demonstrated fibrin deposition in the upper dermis and/or dermo-epidermal junction in 75% of 24 cases of lichen sclerosus, and with indirect immunofluorescence, Dickie et al.[3] found IgM and C_3 present as a linear deposit along the basement membrane. Noting the similarity of lichen sclerosus to some cases of a dermatologic disorder known as morphea, Uitto and his co-workers[21] suggested that immunologic events which stimulate collagen production by dermal fibroblasts may initiate the disease process. At present, an immunologic cause of the disease has not been proven, but these early findings are compatible with the ultrastructural morphologic observations of Mann and Cowan.[16] These investigators found the most pronounced changes in lichen sclerosus to be confined to the dermis and described the passage of degenerate dermal material into the epidermis. Taken altogether, the research findings to date strongly suggest that the basic problem lies with the dermal connective tissue and that the epidermal changes are the secondary results of a deeper process which may have an immunologic basis. As more is learned about the functional changes which occur in the immune system as part of the aging process, this aspect of lichen sclerosus may become more defined.

Hormones are also involved, and untreated postmenopausal women with vulvar lichen sclerosus have decreased levels of plasma dihydrotestosterone. Topical testosterone therapy corrects this deficiency,[9] and the possibility of a local tissue enzyme defect is under investigation.

Finally, genetic factors may also play a role. A total of fifteen families have been identified in which the disease has occurred in succeeding generations.[10,18] Within these families, daughters have tended to acquire the disease at about the same age as did their mothers.

Other disorders of vulvar skin, which become more common with advancing age, include the small one millimeter dark red papules known as "cherry angiomata," the larger and more purple-colored angiokeratomata, and the darkly pigmented and raised lesions of seborrheic keratosis. Long dormant herpes simplex and herpes zoster may recur in the vulvar area and buttocks with chronic immunosuppression. It is the postmenopausal age group in which Paget's disease, squamous carcinoma of the vulva, and carcinoma of the Bartholin gland are most frequently found. A high index of neoplastic suspicion is therefore warranted whenever the aging vulva is examined. Research efforts have now been focused on all aspects of aging. This new impetus is well timed, for many mysteries of the climacteric, including those related to the vulva, still await satisfactory solution.

REFERENCES

1. Bushkell LL, Friedrich EG, and Jordan RE. An appraisal of routine direct immunofluorescence in vulvar disorders. Acta Dermatovener 61:157-161, 1981.
2. Cinberg BL. Postmenopausal pruritus vulvae. Am J Obstet Gynecol 49:647-657, 1945.
3. Dickie RJ, Horne CH, Sutherland HW, Bewsher PD, and Stankler L. Direct evidence of localized immunological damage in vulvar lichen sclerosus. J Clin Pathol 35:1395-1397, 1982.
4. Flynt J and Gallup DG. Childhood lichen sclerosus. Obstet Gynecol 53:79s, 1979.
5. Friedrich EG. Lichen sclerosus. J Reprod Med 17:147-154, 1976.
6. Friedrich EG. *Vulvar Disease*, ed. 2. Philadelphia, WB Saunders, 1983.
7. Friedrich EG. Topical testosterone for benign vulvar dystrophy. Obstet Gynecol 37:667-686, 1971.
8. Friedrich EG, Julian CG, and Woodruff JD. Acridine orange fluorescence in vulvar dysplasia. Am J Obstet Gynecol 90:1281-1287, 1964.
9. Friedrich EG and Kalra PS. Serum levels of sex hormones in vulvar lichen sclerosus, and the effect of topical testosterone. New Engl J Med 310:488-491, 1984.
10. Friedrich EG and MacLaren NK. Genetic aspects of lichen sclerosus. Gynecol, 1984.
11. Harrington CI. An investigation into the incidence of auto-immune disorders in patients with lichen sclerosus et atrophicus. Brit J Dermatol 101 (Suppl. 17):12, 1979.
12. Hart WR, Norris HJ, and Helwig EB. Relation of lichen sclerosus et atrophicus of the vulva to development of carcinoma. Obstet Gynecol 45:369-377, 1975.
13. International Society for the Study of Vulvar Disease. New nomenclature for vulvar disease. Obstet Gynecol 47:122-124, 1976.
14. Jasionowski EA and Jasionowski PA. Further observations on the effect of topical progesterone on vulvar disease. Am J Obstet Gynecol 134:565-567, 1979.

15. Kaufman RH, Gardner HL, Brown D, et al. Vulvar dystrophies: an evaluation. Am J Obstet Gynecol 120:363-367, 1974.
16. Mann PR and Cowan MA. Ultrastructural changes in four cases of lichen sclerosus et atrophicus. Brit J Dermatol 89:223-231, 1973.
17. Mering JH. A surgical approach to intractable pruritus vulvae. Am J Obstet Gynecol 64:619-627, 1952.
18. Murphy FR, Lipa M, and Haberman HF. Familial vulvar dystrophy of lichen sclerosus type. Arch Dermatol 118:329-331, 1982.
19. Nauth HF. Local testosterone treatment of lichen sclerosus of the vulva. Geburtshilfe und Frauenheilkunde 42:476-481, 1982.
20. Rigano A and Mollica G. Histochemistry of some enzyme activities of glucose metabolism in the normal and pathological human vulvar epithelium. Minerva Ginecol 18:1131-1135, 1966.
21. Uitto J, Santa Cruz DJ, Bauer EA, et al. Morphea and lichen sclerosus et atrophicus. J Am Acad Dermatol 3:271-279, 1980.
22. Williams GA, Richardson AC, and Hathcock EW. Topical testosterone in dystrophic diseases of the vulva. Am J Obstet Gynecol 96:21-30, 1966.
23. Woodruff JD and Babaknia A. Local alcohol injection of the vulva. Obstet Gynecol 54:512-514, 1979.
24. Woodruff JD, Borkowf HI, Holzman GB, et al. Metabolic activity in normal and abnormal vulvar epithelia. Am J Obstet Gynecol 91:809-819, 1965.
25. Zelle K. Treatment of vulvar dystrophies with topical testosterone propionate. Am J Obstet Gynecol 109:570-572, 1971.

6

GERIATRIC GYNECOLOGIC ONCOLOGY

C. ROBERT STANHOPE, M.D.

Although approximately 50% of gynecologic cancers occur in women who are more than 65 years of age, relatively little attention has been focused on the special problems created by gynecologic cancer in the geriatric patient.

The overall risk of developing cancer in women between 65 and 85 years of age is 15.5%, in contrast to a risk of 6% in women between 35 and 55 years of age.[1] In addition to this increased risk in the later years, the proportion of women living beyond 65 is steadily increasing, making gynecologic cancer in geriatric patients a major health problem in the United States.

For some gynecologic cancers, the incidence increases with age, although specific differences related to age and race have been noted.[2] For example, the risk of vulvar cancer in white women increases steadily with age while black women have a bimodal age incidence curve. The rates are much higher for black women than for white women younger than 55, but become lower or approximately the same thereafter. The risk of vaginal cancer increases steadily with age in women of both races. The incidence of invasive epidermoid cervical cancer increases more rapidly with age than does that of any other gynecologic cancer, but while it tends to level off after ages 40 or 45 for white women, it increases slowly after that age for black women. Adenocarcinoma of the cervix follows the same pattern but with an approximate 10-year delay. Endometrial cancer in white women has a peak incidence between the ages of 55 and 70 years, after which the incidence decreases. In black women, this decline in incidence in later years is not seen. The incidence of epithelial ovarian cancer increases very slowly but steadily after the age of 55, as does the incidence of sex cord ovarian tumors. Ovarian germ cell tumors, however, have a peak incidence in women less than 30 years of age.

Appropriate initial treatment of women over 65 who have vulvar, endometrial, or ovarian carcinoma involves major surgical intervention, often long periods of anesthesia, and possible significant loss of blood. In comparison, vaginal or cervical cancer is best managed nonsurgically with radiation therapy—either external, or intracavitary or interstitial. Women with endometrial cancer confined to the uterus require a combination of radiation therapy and surgery. Patients with ovarian cancer who undergo tumor reductive surgery are most frequently treated with chemotherapy, which can have inherent major risks to cardiac, renal, neural, and myeloproliferative systems.

In planning the initial treatment for gynecologic cancer, age alone is not a contraindication to vigorous primary treatment. If a pessimistic, conservative approach is advocated, one can expect few responses to treatment and no improved survival rate. Gynecologic oncologists caring for patients who are more than 65 years old must exercise careful pretreatment evaluation, pay close attention to detail, provide essential preoperative medical treatment, and use informed judgment to ensure the best possible results.

This chapter discusses screening and diagnosis, preoperative evaluation, radiation therapy, and chemotherapy as specifically related to the geriatric patient. In addition, appropriate management is outlined for vulvar, vaginal, cervical, endometrial, and ovarian carcinomas.

Screening and Diagnosis

Women over 65 are less responsive to health maintenance programs, especially programs involving the genital tract. Long patient delays are common in elderly women with vulvar cancer or the early symptoms and signs of ovarian carcinoma which are ascribed, all too frequently, to aging and minor gastrointestinal dysfunction.

Yearly gynecologic examination in women over 65 should be strongly encouraged, with careful attention given to the vulva and vagina, where visible or palpable abnormalities must be biopsied, and to the cervix, where Pap smears provide the earliest possible clue to cervical neoplasia. Abnormal uterine bleeding or finding endometrial cells on cervical cytologic study in the postmenopausal woman mandate endometrial sampling. Careful rectovaginal abdominal examinations offer the earliest clues to adnexal pathologic changes. In addition, breast examination, rectal examination, and stool guaiac tests are essential office procedures to screen for breast or colon carcinoma.

Preoperative Evaluation

Generally, surgical procedures are tolerated well by elderly patients because of technological advances that have led to the proper identification of patients at extreme risk and to the proper approach to monitoring patients at moderate risk, especially when appropriate metabolic and cardiopulmonary abnormalities are discovered preoperatively.

To assure that surgery will benefit a patient, a careful and complete history must be taken and a physical examination done just before the proposed surgery. Also important are a complete blood study including platelet count, serum creatinine, serum glutamic–oxalacetic transaminase, lactic acid dehydrogenase, alkaline phosphatase, serum bilirubin, calcium, albumin, total serum proteins, prothrombin time, partial thromboplastin time, fibrinogen, urinalysis, serum electrolytes, and blood urea nitrogen.

Posteroanterior and lateral roentgenograms of the chest should be part of each patient's preoperative evaluation. If pelvic surgery is planned, an intravenous pyelogram should be obtained. Any patient with a history of bowel dysfunction or findings suggestive of an intestinal lesion should have a barium enema study, sigmoidoscopy, and possibly an upper gastrointestinal series. The value of an ultrasound examination of the pelvis or abdomen, when masses are palpable, is questionable. The precise role of computed tomography (CT) for the gynecologic oncologist has not been satisfactorily defined, except as an aid to detect para-aortic nodal or parenchymal hepatic involvement with metastatic cancer. An electrocardiogram should be obtained on all elderly patients and in selected younger patients when pulmonary or cardiac problems exist. Arterial blood gases and pulmonary function studies are also helpful.

A recent study[3] emphasized the value of invasive monitoring techniques in reducing the operative mortality in elderly patients. Of 148 consecutive patients more than 60 years of age evaluated after having been judged as suitable candidates for surgery, only 13.5% had normal hemodynamic, respiratory, and oxygen-transport functions. Mild physiologic abnormalities indicating a very high operative risk were found in 63.5% of the patients. More advanced functional aberrations were found in 23%, and when the latter patients underwent the planned major surgery under general anesthesia in spite of the warning, all died. These authors concluded that invasive preoperative assessment of the elderly patient discloses many serious physiologic abnormalities which, when corrected or when the plans for surgery are altered, can improve the life expectancy of elderly patients undergoing major surgery.

Radiation Therapy

Radiation treatment is sometimes modified for psychotic patients or patients with coexisting carcinoma; however, other medical conditions commonly seen in elderly patients, such as hypertension, diabetes, or cardiopulmonary diseases, rarely are contraindications for radiation therapy unless the diseases are severe. Age is not a limiting factor for radiation therapy; however, chronic inflammatory bowel conditions such as diverticulitis may exacerbate after pelvic irradiation. Furthermore, quiescent pelvic inflammatory disease in an elderly patient may flare up and cause severe peritonitis and even death from sepsis.

Chemotherapy

Chemotherapists tend to individualize the treatment of elderly patients, especially patients more than 80 years of age. While there are no specific age-related complications or adverse reactions to chemotherapy, some elderly patients cannot tolerate aggressive combination chemotherapy without major morbidity. Also, some elderly patients dictate, to a certain extent, the degree of therapy they wish to have and may choose either less or more aggressive forms of chemotherapy. Elderly patients are frequently less attentive to details, and explicit instructions must be given not only to the patient but also to family members so that accidents in the administration of drugs do not occur. Additional attention must also be given to the nutritional needs or metabolic alterations that seem to occur earlier in elderly patients who experience intense nausea, vomiting, or diarrhea.

Management of Specific Cancers

Vulvar Carcinoma. Carcinoma of the vulva usually occurs in women who are past middle age; in fact, 52% are more than 65 years old.[4] Frequently, these women have other conditions such as cardiac, metabolic, or pulmonary disorders for which adjustments must be made in the overall plan of treatment. These elderly women, despite their age and frequent associated medical problems, tolerate vulvar surgery with ease, experiencing few major life-threatening complications. For this reason, age alone should not be considered a deterrent to the appropriate surgical approach for vulvar carcinoma. Prophylactic heparin and antibiotics have proved to be very useful.

Carcinoma-in-situ of the vulva is considered to be a multifocal process, and while a very conservative approach of local excision and close follow-up has been taken in younger women, total excision of the vulva in the geriatric patient is most appropriate, particularly when orgasmic sexual function is not a major concern of the patient.

The treatment for microinvasive vulvar carcinoma must be individualized, based upon the volume and extent of the microinvasive process. Radical vulvectomy is appropriate for patients with lesions less than 1 cm in diameter, while radical vulvectomy with inguinal lymphadenectomy is indicated for patients with larger or more extensive lesions.

The standard surgical procedure for invasive vulvar carcinoma is radical vulvectomy and bilateral inguinal lymphadenectomy. In certain patients, unilateral or bilateral pelvic lymphadenectomy may be required. These include patients with metastatic involvement of Cloquet's node, a primary carcinoma of the Bartholin gland, or a nonsuperficial melanoma of the vulva. A new approach currently under investigation is not to perform pelvic lymphadenectomy but to treat the external and common iliac lymph nodes and perhaps the lower para–aortic lymph nodes with external radiation therapy. This approach should decrease the operative time and postoperative morbidity, that is, decrease lymphocysts, wound necrosis, and leg edema, which occur more frequently when pelvic lymphadenectomy is performed with radical vulvectomy.

Vaginal Carcinoma. Carcinoma-in-situ of the vaginal apex after hysterectomy can be locally destroyed effectively using a CO_2 laser, or it can be surgically removed by partial vaginectomy. The latter approach is advised for patients who have had previous irradiation to the pelvis.

Patients with invasive vaginal carcinoma are best treated with a combination of external and intracavitary or interstitial radiation. Specific treatment is tailored to the location and size of the lesion. Obliteration of the vaginal canal can be expected after radiation therapy. To help preserve the vaginal canal, the regular use of a smooth plastic dilator or frequent sexual intercourse is the best the physician can suggest.

Cervical Carcinoma. Both dysplasia and carcinoma-in-situ should be eradicated when discovered in elderly patients. Local destruction by the use of CO_2 laser or cryotherapy can be considered; however, conization or hysterectomy may be necessary.

Patients with early invasive cervical carcinoma can be treated with radical surgery or radiation, with similar survival expectations. In elderly patients, irradiation is considered the most appropriate treatment, and combinations of external and intracavitary irradiation using modern techniques are generally well tolerated regardless of age, except when diverticulitis or chronic pelvic inflammatory disease is present.

Endometrial Carcinoma. The age of a patient at the time of a diagnosis of endometrial carcinoma is of prognostic significance, because younger patients have a more favorable prognosis.[5] In one study,[6] the 5-year survival rate in patients who were more than 70 years old was 60.9%, compared with 92.1% for patients between the ages of 40 and 49 years. However, 79% of the younger patients had the tumor confined to the uterine corpus, compared with 62% in the group more than 70 years old. Furthermore, superficial invasion of the myometrium was present in 76% of the younger patients but in only 43% of the older patients. These facts lead to the conclusion that, while age is a related factor, age alone does not mean a less favorable outcome in older patients, although elderly patients tend to have more extensive involvement of the uterus.

The current management of endometrial carcinoma is individualized, depending on the stage and grade of involvement, as well as the size of the uterus. Abdominal or vaginal hysterectomy with bilateral salpingo–oophorectomy may be sufficient therapy for clinical stage I-A, grade 1 lesions, providing pathologic examination does not uncover (1) a higher grade endometrial carcinoma, (2) endocervical or ovarian involvement, or (3) myometrial invasion. If one of these is discovered, external irradiation or vaginal brachytherapy (or both) would be indicated postoperatively.

Where the uterine canal is less than 8 cm long and when only grade 1 or grade 2 cancer is present, intracavitary irradiation followed by abdominal or vaginal hysterectomy with bilateral adnexectomy is appropriate. Again, pathologic assessment may indicate the need for postoperative external irradiation.

In most other stage I or stage II endometrial cancers, preoperative external and intracavitary irradiation, followed in six weeks by abdominal hysterectomy and bilateral adnexectomy, is considered standard therapy.

Treatment for clinical stage III or stage IV endometrial carcinoma must be individualized, employing possibly surgery, radiation therapy, chemotherapy, and hormonal therapy (Table 1).

In patients with endometrial cancer, who are considered inoperable for medical reasons, sophisticated intracavitary therapy alone or in conjunction with external irradiation appears to provide better rates of uterine control than does external irradiation alone.[7]

Ovarian Carcinoma.   Minimal treatment for the elderly patient with ovarian carcinoma should be the removal of both ovaries and the uterus. Removal of as much tumor as possible is considered optimal and should be attempted whenever the medical condition of the patient permits. Obviously, there are situations when the extent of disease, the poor nutrition of the patient, or other medical problems will not permit this approach. A more conservative surgical approach must be taken

TABLE 1.   TREATMENT PLAN FOR ENDOMETRIAL CANCER

Stage	Grade	Treatment
I-A	1	Abdominal or vaginal hysterectomy and bilateral salpingo-oophorectomy (BSO)
I-A	2	Intracavitary radiation; abdominal or vaginal hysterectomy and BSO
I-B (small uterus)	1-2	Intracavitary radiation; abdominal or vaginal hysterectomy and BSO
I-B (large uterus)	1-2	External radiation plus intracavitary radiation; abdominal hysterectomy and BSO
I-A–I-B	3	External radiation plus intracavitary radiation; abdominal hysterectomy and BSO
II	1-2-3	External radiation plus intracavitary radiation; abdominal hysterectomy and BSO
III-IV	. . .	Individualized treatment: radiation therapy, surgery, chemotherapy, hormonal therapy

in these situations, and subsequent expectations of chemotherapy must be realistically limited as well to palliation and control of effusion.

A definite philosophy for the surgical technique has been established. The primary surgical exploration of a patient of any age who is suspected of having ovarian cancer requires a long midline incision extending from the symphysis pubis to a point 5 cm above the umbilicus. This incision enables the surgeon to explore the entire abdominal cavity. A Pfannenstiel incision is inadequate and should not be used.

After exploration of the pelvis and abdomen, removal of the largest tumor mass is attempted first. Most often, ovarian cancer can be dissected from serosal surfaces with minimal damage to underlying structures. For example, masses can be resected from the small intestine, colon, abdominal wall, liver, or diaphragm. Sometimes, a segment of small intestine or colon needs to be resected. Generally, only one segment is removed.

Tumor involving the terminal ileum and cecum may require resection and an anastomosis between the ilium and the ascending colon. Tumor extensively involving and invading the rectosigmoid colon may require resection of the colonic lesion with the proximal colonic limb brought out as an end-colostomy and the rectum oversewn. Recent technical advances with stapling instruments make it possible to safely complete end-to-end inverting anastomoses in the distal intestinal tract, thus avoiding colostomy in some situations when the distal rectosigmoid is resected.

Even if dense cancer involves the porta hepatis or regions above the superior mesenteric artery or the lesser omentum and surgical reduction is limited, patients still benefit from the removal of large masses that may be causing pressure on the bladder, the rectosigmoid colon, or the pelvic veins. These patients will have improved urinary tract or gastrointestinal function even though they may not survive as long as patients who have no residual or unresected cancer after primary surgery.

Currently, chemotherapy is the most effective postoperative treatment for ovarian cancer. Combinations of drugs that have proven to be individually effective appear to achieve better results than single-drug therapy. The drugs most active in inducing responses in ovarian cancer are cyclophosphamide, hexamethylmelamine, doxorubicin, and cisplatin.

After at least 12 courses of chemotherapy, a "second-look" operation can be performed to assess a patient's status and to plan future treatment.

Conclusion

Elderly women are at greater risk for developing genital malignancies and require careful pretreatment evaluations and individualized therapy based on the volume and extent of the disease. Coexisting medical factors must be considered, however, and age alone should not be the criterion on which treatment is based.

REFERENCES

1. Seidman, H., Silverberg, E., Bodden, A. Probabilities of eventually developing and of dying of cancer (risk among persons previously undiagnosed with the cancer). CA: A Cancer Journal for Clinicians 28:33–46, 1978.
2. Berg, J.W., Lampe, J.G. High-risk factors in gynecologic cancer. Cancer 48:429–441, 1981.
3. Del Guercio, L.R.M., Cohn, J.D. Monitoring operative risk in the elderly. JAMA 243:1350–1355, 1980.
4. Green, T.H., Jr., Ulfelder, H., Meigs, J.V. Epidermoid carcinoma of the vulva: an analysis of 238 cases. Part I. Etiology and diagnosis. Am. J. Obstet. Gynecol. 75:834–847, 1958.
5. Sall, S., Sonnenblick, B., Stone, M.L. Factors affecting survival of patients with endometrial adenocarcinoma. Am. J. Obstet. Gynecol. 107:116–123, 1970.
6. Nilsen, P.A., Koller, O. Carcinoma of the endometrium in Norway 1957–1960 with special reference to treatment results. Am. J. Obstet. Gynecol. 105:1099–1109, 1969.
7. Landgren, R.C., Fletcher, G.H., Delclos, L., Wharton, J.T. Irradiation of endometrial cancer in patients with medical contraindication to surgery or with unresectable lesions. Am. J. Roentgen. 126:148–154, 1976.

7

POSTMENOPAUSAL BLEEDING

MURRAY JOSEPH CASEY, M.D., FACOG, FACS

Postmenopausal bleeding has long been considered a grave sign, at one time associated with more than a 50% incidence of neoplastic disease.[1-3] Because of greater patient awareness and closer opportunities for physician surveillance, this symptom has heralded the presence of genital cancer proportionately less frequently during recent years.[4-9] At the Mount Sinai Medical Center in Milwaukee from 1975 through 1979, invasive cancers were discovered in only 13% of 233 postmenopausal women who underwent diagnostic D&C for genital bleeding.[9] Nevertheless, as a possible warning of underlying malignancy, postmenopausal bleeding remains an important signal which demands expeditious evaluation. Although the American literature up to 1950 indicated a 50:50 ratio of cervical and lower genital tract cancers to uterine corpus tumors, mainly endometrial adenocarcinomas, in postmenopausal bleeders,[2-7] a much lower proportion of cervical cancer was diagnosed among predominantly Jewish populations in the United States and Israel.[10,11] More recently, the decreasing incidence of invasive cervical neoplasms in North America has led to less frequent reports of these tumors being the cause of postmenopausal bleeding in general.[8] The uterine cervix was found to be the primary site for only 2 of the 30 malignancies diagnosed following examination and D&C for postmenopausal bleeding in a more heterogenous population at Mount Sinai Medical Center in Milwaukee than the Jewish population reported in Jerusalem.[9,11] Besides greater heterogeneity of the population served in Milwaukee, virtually all of the patients evaluated for postmenopausal bleeding at Mount Sinai Medical Center had previously been examined by a trained gynecologist prior to their hospital admission.[9]

Endocrinology Of The Menopause

Before discussing the pathology associated with postmenopausal bleeding, it is important to define and briefly review the endocrine physiology of the female reproductive system through the course of midlife.

Ovarian Cycle and Hormonal Response. During the reproductive years, cyclic monthly fluctuations of delicately balanced circulating estrogens and superimposed progesterone of ovarian origin (Fig. 7:1) stimulate and maintain endometrial proliferation, buildup, maturation and secretion.

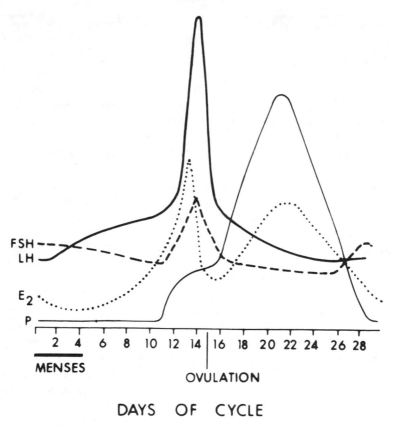

Figure 7:1. Monthly fluctuation of circulating estrogen (E_2), progesterone (P) and gonadotrophins (LH and FSH) during a characteristic ovulatory cycle in the premenopausal woman. (Conn. Med. 41:776, 1977, reprinted with permission.)

Upon a failure to conceive, it is the withdrawal of this hormonal support from the endometrium which leads to menstruation. In the ovulatory female, development of the ovarian Graafian follicle takes place in response to the gonadotrophins, follicle stimulating hormone (FSH) and luteinizing hormone (LH), which are released from the pituitary gland under control of the hypothalamus. Estradiol ($E2$) originating in ovarian follicles, has been shown to be the major component of the circulating serum estrogen pool throughout the reproductive years[12]; although small amounts of estrogenic hormones, mainly estrone (E1), are contributed by metabolic conversion of androgens produced in the adrenal glands and ovaries.[13] Following cessation of regular monthly ovulation during the fifth and sixth decades of life, the ovary no longer is capable of this cyclic secretory response to pituitary gonadotrophin stimulation because of the absence of maturing Graafian follicles. Menopause is simply that time in a woman's middle adult life when the last functional menstrual period marks the termination of ovulation and thus the end of her reproductive capacity.

Postmenopausal Hormonal Milieu. Menopause may occur abruptly, or ovulation and menstruation may become less frequent over several months or even years. When extended intervals of anovulation occur during this time, they are usually and normally manifest by months of oligomenorrhea. Finally, permanent ovarian failure is recognized by the enduring amenorrhea which follows menopause. Spontaneous ovulation can take place after many months of ovulatory inactivity in the perimenopausal period; however, ovulation after more than 12 months of amenorrhea is most unusual and difficult to document.[4,6,14] Therefore, by convention, uterine bleeding which occurs more than one year beyond the last menstrual period during the climacteric is defined as "postmenopausal bleeding."[4]

During prolonged intervals of anovulation and following the menopause, estrone (E1) is the major estrogenic component of the serum. This steroid is the product of end organ conversion of androstenedione (A), secreted in large part by the adrenal gland, although the ovary, stimulated by gonadotrophins, is capable of producing this as well as other androgens.[13,15-19] Subcutaneous adipose tissues and the liver have been identified as sites in which the active conversion of A to E1 takes place[17-19] (Fig. 7:2). In the absence of ovulation, there is loss of the ovarian-hypothalamic-pituitary feedback mechanism which characterizes and controls follicular development during monthly ovulatory cycles. Inability of the polycystic and postmenopausal ovary to respond to gonadotrophin stimulation by normal follicular development, ovulation and secretion of E2 and progesterone results in persistence of markedly elevated plasma levels of LH and FSH in the hypothalamic-pituitary effort to override an

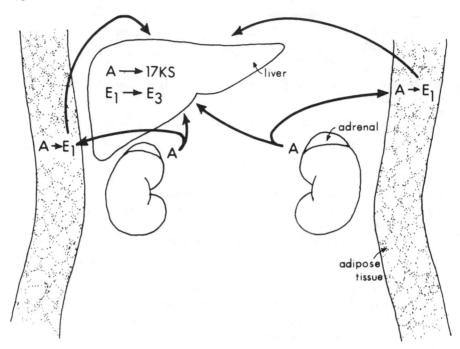

Figure 7:2. Estrogen production following menopause proceeds mainly from conversion of androstenedione (A) to estrone (E_1) in adipose tissues. Adrenal synthesis is the major source of A. Androstenedione and E_1 are metabolized in the liver to 17-ketosteroid (17-KS) and estriol (E_3) excretory products of low biologic activity. (Conn. Med. 41:776, 1977, reprinted with permission.)

unresponsive ovary (Fig. 7:3). A period of oligoovulation which which typifies the premenopausal years of some women and the waning ovarian function in the early postmenopausal period are characterized by a state of "persistent estrus" in which low levels of plasma estrogens are associated with high levels of pituitary gonadotrophins. With continued aging, there is usually a gradual decline in glandular secretin of androstenedione; so while metabolic conversion of A to E1 may become more efficient in some women with aging,[18] lower production of A results in a general tendency to diminishing levels of E1 with advanced age.[20]

Endometrium Following Menopause

After menopause and during periods of anovulation, endometrial maturation, completed under stimulation of E1 and progesterone from the follicular ovary, and menstrual

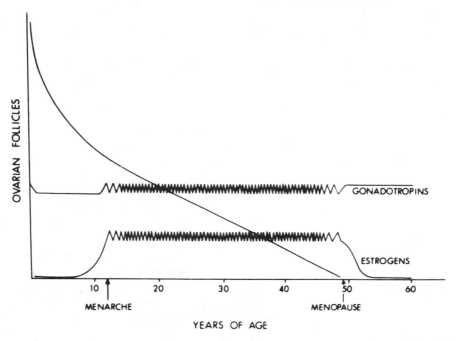

Figure 7:3. Pituitary gonadotrophins (LH and FSH) circulate at inverse proportion to the biological levels of estrogens, primarily estradiol (E_2) during each ovarian cycle which typifies the normally ovulatory reproductive period of adult female life. LH and FSH are high prior to menarche and following ovarian follicle exhaustion after menopause. Estrone (E_1), the predominant estrogen after follicular atresia, may persist at low nonfluctuating levels after menopause.

sloughing, which takes place upon hormonal withdrawal at the end of each monthly cycle, can no longer occur.

Atrophic Endometrium. Ordinarily, the levels of circulating estrogen following menopause are insufficient to cause significant endometrial proliferation and growth. Atrophic endometrium with inactive, quiescent glands of diminished number and stromal dominance is the rule. Sometimes, endometrial biopsies taken after the menopause will show areas of cystic atrophy with multiple small dilated glands surrounded by inactive-appearing stroma. An exaggeration of this endometrial pattern may be seen in an endocrine milieu of continuous uninterrupted estrogen, when under this stimulation multiple endometrial gland luminae may become so dilated that they take on a cystic configuration and begin to constrict and crowd intervening stroma. This pattern, reminiscent of Swiss cheese when seen on histology slides, has been termed "cystic glandular hyperplasia." These tissues are unstable and prone to break down.

Adenomatous Hyperplasia and Adenocarcinoma. The development of proliferative endometrial hyperplasia has been associated with a hormonal milieu of "persistent estrus" from endogenous sources, such as anovulatory polycystic ovaries and estrogen-secreting tumors, and from exogenous sources, such as therapeutic estrogens.[19] This "adenomatous hyperplasia" may be focal or diffuse. In the course of hyperplastic proliferation, intraluminal cellular crowding results in a pattern of pseudostratification with nuclei lying in adjacent cells at different levels in order to be accommodated within the densely packed glands. The most severe forms of adenomatous hyperplasia are characterized by intraluminal budding and papillary growth; and interglandular stroma may be so compressed by the hyperplastic epithelial tissues that the abnormal glands seem to lie back to back. This lesion is believed to be a precursor of endometrial adenocarcinoma.[19,21] When nuclear atypia is present, some authorities have termed this extreme variety, "atypical hyperplasia" or endometrial carcinoma *in situ.*

The close association of adenomatous hyperplasia with frankly invasive endometrial carcinoma has long been recognized.[2,19] Indeed, a common etiologic factor is implied by the frequent coexistence of hyperplastic changes of the endometrium with endometrial adenocarcinoma.[19,21] In the spectrum of development, malignant transformation is marked by cellular atypia and glandular proliferation progressing until there is finally invasion of the endometrial stroma. In the earliest forms of endometrial carcinoma, glandular architecture is generally preserved. Dedifferentiation and irregular growth leads to the development of solid areas of tumor and ultimately the loss of glandular structure. For prognostic purposes, the International Federation of Gynecologists and Obstetricians has recommended the grading of endometrial carcinomas as: *G1* highly differentiated adenocarcinoma; *G2* differentiated adenomatous carcinoma with partially solid areas; and *G3* predominantly solid or entirely undifferentiated carcinoma.

Risk Factors for Endometrial Carcinoma

Substantial evidence has accumulated linking the development of endometrial hyperplasia and an increased risk for endometrial carcinoma with those conditions which result in exposure of the endometrium to higher than usual levels of noncyclic estrogen unopposed by intermittent progesterone stimulation.[19,21]

Acyclic Ovarian Hormones. Long periods of anovulation in patients with polycystic ovaries are associated with increased production of ovarian androgens and thence their conversion through androstenedione to estrone without the fluctuating levels of estradiol and progesterone, which are seen in women with normally functioning follicular ovaries. Characteristically, these patients will have elevated levels of serum LH which can be suppressed by the administration of progestins.[22] Although fewer than 3% of endometrial carcinomas are diagnosed in women younger than 40 years of age, an incidence of endometrial cancer as high as 20% has been reported in young women with polycystic ovary syndrome.[23] Furthermore, 20-30% of postmenopausal women with estrogen-secreting ovarian tumors of the granulosa-theca-lutein group have been found to have coincidental endometrial carcinomas.[19,24]

Exogenous Estrogens. Abundant reports point to the association of therapeutically administered exogenous estrogens with the development of endometrial carcinoma. Although endometrial cancer is extremely rare or nonexistent in patients with gonadal dysgenesis (Turner's syndrome), there are several observations of this neoplasm developing in young people who had been treated with estrogenic medications to induce maturation of the secondary sexual characteristics.[19,25] In addition, estrogens in the form of sequential contraceptive medications in which there were relatively high estrogen to progesterone ratios have been implicated as etiologic factors in the development of endometrial carcinomas in young women who used these birth control methods.[19,26] In 1975, two epidemiologic studies pointed out that a significantly greater number of patients with endometrial cancer had previously been treated with exogenous estrogens for menopausal symptoms than had their matched cohorts.[27,28] Subsequent reports confirmed an increased risk for the development of endometrial carcinoma in those women who used these drugs. However, it now appears that this risk may be minimized or eliminated by adding exogenous progestins to the regimen during the last half of each monthly cycle in which estrogens are administered.[29] These observations were especially interesting in view of earlier reports that some cases of severe adenomatous hyperplasia could be reversed and matured to normal endometrium by the cyclic use of estrogen-progestin medications.[30]

Increased Androgenic Conversion. In the absence of exogenous estrogens and identifiable endogenous estrogen sources, the development of endometrial cancer among the young may belong almost exclusively to the realm of those with marked obesity.[31] Between 1971 and 1977 only 3 of 176 women first treated at New Britain General Hospital in Connecticut for endometrial cancers were diagnosed while younger than 40 years of age.[31] The respective weights of these patients ranged from 220 and 270 to 325 pounds. Although about half of those who develop endometrial cancer in the perimenopausal or postmenopausal period are classifiably overweight, depending upon various criteria, these tumors do occur in other women who are not obese and who have had no history of oligoovulation during their reproductive years.

There is experimental evidence that adipose tissues from some women with endometrial cancer may more efficiently convert A to E1, *in vitro*.[17] Thus it appears that a state of persistent estrus can result through increased production of E1 from A in either a "larger factory," as seen in obesity,[18] or a "more efficient factory," as in the latter women.[17] Both E1 and its precursor androgens are normally metabolized to excretory products in the healthy liver; so hepatic dysfunctions caused by cirrhosis or fatty infiltration, as might occur in obese patients, may further contribute to elevated, noncyclic levels of circulating estrogens.

Other Factors. The significance of dietary habits has yet to be elucidated, especially with regard to foods which are high in cholesterol and the acetate precursors that form the steroid nucleus on which endogenous sex hormones are built. The importance of genetic predispositions to obesity and endometrial cancer also invites further exploration. Diabetes mellitus and high blood pressure frequently accompany obesity and occur with unusual frequency in women with endometrial cancer. This could be due only to their obesity or may reflect a common underlying heritable endocrinopathy. Epidemiologic studies have implicated both family and a past personal history of cancer, especially arising in the breast or genitalia, as increasing the risk for developing endometrial carcinoma.[19]

High levels of serum LH, as seen in anovulatory and postmenopausal conditions, have been reported in patients with both hypothyroid and hyperthyroid conditions; it is of interest that some form of thyroidopathy or treatment with thyroid hormone was reported by about 9% of patients diagnosed with endometrial carcinoma at the New Britain General Hospital in Connecticut,[31] and that 10% of women with endometrial cancer at Mount Sinai Medical Center in Milwaukee reported the use of thyroid medications.[9] This would seem high; however, no data are available to compare these figures with the incidence of thyroid dysfunction in the population of women from which those patients were drawn.

Differential Diagnosis of Postmenopausal Bleeding

After appropriate investigation to rule out potential extragenital sources of hemorrhage such as hematuria, per rectal bleeding, etc., the lower genital tract is examined to document the presence or absence of lesions which might contribute to a presenting symptom of postmenopausal bleeding. Such causes are usually obvious on inspection, but may require the aid of screening cytology and colposcopy for detection.

Lower Genital Tract: Brewer and Miller found that only 5% of their patients in Chicago during the 1940's and early 1950's were admitted in order to distinguish between uterine and other sources of postmenopausal bleeding.[4] In general, other authors reported that 8-12% of the postmenopausal patients reviewed by them had lower tract sites of bleeding.[2,3,5-8] Carcinomas and sarcomas of the vulva and vagina, including malignant melanomas, frequently present as genital bleeding, although such tumors account for only a small proportion of patients with postmenopausal bleeding.[11,32,33] Other recognized sites of postmenopausal contact bleeding from the lower gential tract are urethral caruncles and prolapse, inflammatory lesions and benign tumors of the vulva and vagina, and trauma of the vaginal mucosa from prolapse, pessaries or coitus.[2-8] Trauma to lower tract lesions may result in postcoital hemorrhage, or spontaneous spotting and bleeding may be experienced. The senile atrophic vagina is particularly susceptible to minor trauma from infection and sexual manipulations.

Uterine Cervix: Cervical lesions accounted for 20-40% of postmenopausal bleeding reported by authors of the 1950's and before.[2-6] Although large ulcers and exophytic tumors of the uterine cervix are often evident, more subtle cervical pathology, such as minute endocervical polyps and chronic cervicitis, also can be responsible for postcoital bleeding when traumatized. Furthermore, infiltrating cervical epidermoid carcinomas, adenocarcinomas and sarcomas may present as spontaneous or postcoital bleeding after menopause. While malignant cervical tumors were responsible for the majority of postmenopausal bleeding from the uterine cervix in American women prior to the 1950's,[2,3] this was not an important cause among populations with lower incidences of cervical carcinoma.[10,11] Twenty-six of the 233 well-screened patients undergoing examination with anesthesia and D&C for postmenopausal bleeding at Mount Sinai Medical Center in Milwaukee during 1975-1979 were found to have cervical lesions.[9] This included 18 patients with cervical polyps, 2 with severe chronic cervicitis, 4 with cervical intraepithelial neoplasia and 2 with invasive squamous cell carcinomas. Over half (15/26) of these cervical lesions had been noted during the preadmission examination or had been detected on suspicious or positive Pap smears. While the majority of cervical lesions are detected in the outpatient by inspection and cytology, the frequent occurrence of associated pathology in women with postmenopausal bleeding mandates a still more thorough evaluation. Although postmenopausal bleeding was attributable primarily to cervical pathology in only 6% of the Mount Sinai Medical Center series of 233 patients, it is noteworthy that in 9 cases, the cervical lesions were neoplastic or associated with other genital cancers. Furthermore, benign cervical polyps in this series were associated with 2 uterine sarcomas, 1 ovarian carcinoma and 1 *in situ* carcinoma of the cervix. One woman with a class IV Pap smear was found to have both cervical intraepithelial neoplasia and adenocarcinoma of the endometrium. Coexisting endometrial polyps were discovered in 2 of 4 patients with intraepithelial neoplasia and in 4 of 18 patients with cervical polyps. It is therefore important to emphasize that the presence of a lower genital tract or cervical lesion does not preclude the coexistence of an intrauterine source of bleeding. Discovery of such a lesion should not lessen the suspicion of additional uterine or adnexal pathology.

Uterine Corpus: A uterine corpus source was found in over 40% of the women investigated for postmenopausal bleeding before the 1950's.[2-6] Table 1 summarizes the established causes of postmenopausal bleeding in six series from the United States and one from Israel.[2-6,8,11] When lower genital tract and cervical sites are eliminated, it can be seen that endometrial pathology is the predominant factor. The importance of establishing the etiology of uterine bleeding following the menopause can readily be appreciated by noting that in these older series, endometrial malignancies were as often responsible as were benign conditions.

Hyperplasia. The earlier series of patients with post-menopausal bleeding reported endometrial hyperplasia in fewer than 5% and polyps in only 2-9% of the women undergoing D&C. However, in patients evaluated for postmenopausal bleeding at Mount Sinai Medical Center during the late 1970's, 13% were found to have endometrial hyperplasias, and endometrial polyps were discovered in 21%.[9] It is believed that the 1970's represented the peak period of therapeutic estrogen use in this country without superimposed exogenous progestins. A history of significant recent or concurrent estrogen use was obtained in 42% (98/233) of those women who were admitted to Mount Sinai Medical Center for evaluation of postmenopausal bleeding. Endometrial hyperplasia was diagnosed in 26 of the 233 patients in the Mount Sinai series: 19 cases were of the adenomatous variety, and 5 of these were felt to be histologically atypical. It is striking that 79% of the patients with adenomatous hyperplasia gave a history of estrogen use; while only 1 of 5 patients with cystic hyperplasia was known to have used these drugs, albeit no significance is implied.

Polyps. Endometrial polyps are of three types: *Functional polyps* are those which show proliferative or secretory glandular response compatible with the phase of the normal reproductive ovarian cycle, and therefore this type of polyp is very uncommon or nonexistent in the truly postmenopausal woman. *Adenomyomatous polyps* are simply polypoid projections of submucous fibroids enveloped in endometrial tissues which are usually atrophic during the postmenopausal period. Functional and adenomyomatous polyps do not often cause abnormal bleeding unless they prolapse through the cervix or outstrip their blood supply and undergo infarction and necrosis. These two types of polyps are usually discovered only incidentally following hysterectomy for unrelated problems. On the other hand, *hyperplastic polyps* may show any or all stages of the spectrum from "Swiss cheese" cystic hyperplasia to proliferative hyperplasia and finally severely atypical adenomatous hyperplasia. While on histologic review, it is important not to over-interpret as adenocarcinoma the closely packed glands which may occur in some endometrial polyps. It must be borne in mind that invasive neoplasms can coexist with hyperplastic polyps in as many as 15% of the cases.[34] So caution must reign when functional or hyperplastic changes, indicating the likelihood of estrogen

TABLE I. SOURCES OF POSTMENOPAUSAL BLEEDING

Authors (reference)

Year (no. cases reported)

	Taylor & Millen (2) 1938 (406)	Jones & Cantor (3) 1951 (214)	Brewer & Miller (4) 1954 (222)	Woodruff, et al. (5) 1958 (574)	Payne, et al. (6) 1959 (698)	Hawwa, et al. (8) 1970 (335)	Brzezinsky & Bromberg (11) 1953 (187)
Lower genital tract	46 (11%)	17 (8%)	11 (5%)	52 (9%)	86 (12%)	40 (12%)	20 (11%)
Vulva	11 (3%)		3 (1%)	7 (1%)		4 (1%)	1 (<1%)
Malignant	7 (2%)		1 (<1%)	1 (<1%)			1 (<1%)
Benign	4 (<1%)		2 (<1%)	6 (1%)		4 (1%)	
Vagina	35 (9%)	17 (8%)	8 (4%)	45 (8%)		36 (11%)	19 (10%)
Malignant	9 (2%)	1 (<1%)				3 (<1%)	2* (1%)
Benign	26 (7%)	16 (8%)	8 (4%)	45 (8%)		33 (10%)	17 (9%)
Inflammation	11 (3%)	4 (2%)	5 (2%)		42 (6%)		13 (7%)
Prolapse	15 (4%)	8 (4%)					
Pessary		4 (2%)					4 (2%)
Cervix	158 (39%)	74 (35%)	53 (24%)	90 (16%)	248 (36%)	36 (11%)	36 (19%)
Neoplastic	125 (31%)	60 (28%)	24 (11%)	34 (6%)	64 (9%)	14 (4%)	
Squamous ca.			20 (9%)			13 (4%)	
Adenocarcinoma			4 (2%)			1 (<1%)	
Benign	33 (8%)	14 (7%)	29 (13%)	56 (10%)	184 (26%)	22 (7%)	36 (19%)
Inflammation	18 (4%)		12 (5%)			8 (3%)	16 (9%)
Polyp	15 (4%)	14 (7%)	18 (8%)			14 (4%)	20 (11%)
Corpus	167 (41%)	108 (51%)	67 (30%)	201 (35%)	281 (40%)	169 (51%)	113 (60%)
Malignant	106 (26%)	65 (30%)	29 (13%)	53 (9%)	131 (19%)	45 (13%)	13 (7%)
Endometrial ca.	101 (25%)	62 (29%)	27 (12%)			42 (12%)	13 (7%)
Sarcoma	5 (1%)	3 (1%)	2 (<1%)			3 (1%)	
Hyperplastic	11 (3%)	9 (4%)	11 (5%)		19 (3%)	11 (3%)	20 (11%)

Benign	50 (12%)	34 (16%)	27 (12%)	148 (26%)	131 (19%)	113 (34%)	80 (43%)
Myoma	28 (7%)	7 (3%)	8 (4%)			1 (<1%)	17 (9%)
Endomet. polyp	9 (2%)	10 (5%)	19 (9%)			23 (7%)	9 (5%)
Endometritis	7 (2%)	6 (3%)					19 (10%)
"Estrogens"					56 (8%)	89 (27%)	
Atrophic		11 (5%)					35 (19%)
Tube							
Malignant	2 (<1%)		1 (<1%)			1 (<1%)	
Benign	2 (<1%)		1 (<1%)			1 (<1%)	
Ovary		10 (5%)					10 (5%)
Malignant	23 (6%)		6 (3%)	9 (2%)	4 (<1%)	3 (<1%)	5 (3%)
Functional	12 (3%)		4 (2%)	6 (1%)	4 (<1%)		1 (<1%)
Carcinoma	4 (<1%)		1 (<1%)		2 (<1%)	3 (<1%)	3 (2%)
Metastatic	8 (2%)		3 (1%)		2 (<1%)		1 (<1%)
Benign	11 (3%)		2 (<1%)	3 (<1%)			5 (3%)

*includes 2 patients with malignant melanoma

stimulation, are found in any endometrial tissues recovered by curettage for postmenopausal uterine bleeding. Benign endometrial polyps were found in 49 of the 233 patients with postmenopausal bleeding evaluated in Milwaukee at Mount Sinai Medical Center.[9] Four of these patients also had cervical polyps. A further 3 patients had endometrial polyps with areas of atypical hyperplasia. Exogenous estrogens had been recently used by 45% of the patients with endometrial polyps in the Mount Sinai series. Many endometrial adenocarcinomas recovered by curettage show polypoid projections, and one papillary-type carcinoma was discovered among the 22 patients with endometrial cancers in the Mount Sinai series of postmenopausal bleeders.[9]

Carcinoma. Endometrial carcinomas may occur in the postmenopause as purely glandular tumors or with various admixtures of benign or malignant squamous elements. In our review of 159 patients with endometrial carcinomas admitted to New Britain General Hospital over a 7-year period (1971-1977), we could find no apparent relationship between the use of estrogenic medications and the presence or absence of squamous elements.[31,35] It is not the purpose of this discussion to dwell upon the histologic types of endometrial cancer and their implications for treatment or prognosis. However, it should be noted that a favorable outlook for long-term survival with standard therapy of endometrial adenocarcinomas rests primarily on the degree of differentiation of the glandular elements when the tumors are first diagnosed.[36-40] Our observations show clearly that those patients in the Connecticut series who were relatively young when their endometrial carcinomas were diagnosed, had better differentiated tumors.[31] Furthermore, tumors in these younger women were more often still confined to the uterine corpus, and they experienced better survival rates than those women whose endometrial cancers were first discovered beyond the age of 60 years.[35] While the younger patients more frequently reported the use of exogenous estrogen replacement therapy, no conclusion could be drawn from the available data as to whether these medications served as uncovering agents through promotion of symptomatic bleeding, or whether estrogenic medications were important etiologic factors in the early development of this disease.[31,35] Overall, 30.8% of the patients with endometrial carcinoma at New Britain General Hospital had taken estrogens, a figure comparable to estrogen use by 31.8% of postmenopausal women found to have endometrial cancer at Mount Sinai Medical Center.[9,31]

Estrogens. In a study of endometrial biopsies taken from 363 women with postmenopausal bleeding followed in the large Menopause Clinic at Wilford Hall U.S. Air Force Medical Center between 1972 and 1973, Gambrell reported that one-third showed hyperplasia or adenocarcinoma, one-third showed proliferative endometrium and one-third were atrophic.[14] Of course, no polyps were recovered with the biopsy technique which was used. While 46% of the Wilford Hall patients were receiving estrogens for postmenopausal symptoms, only 3 were found to have frank adenocarcinoma on the endometrial biopsy at the time of these studies; 10.7% had adenomatous hyperplasia, and 21.2% had other forms of hyperplasia.[14] Secretory endometrium, as evidence of ovulation, was seen in only 1.9% of these patients and did not occur beyond the age of 55 years.[14] In 233 patients at Mount Sinai Medical Center studied with D&C for postmenopausal bleeding during 1975 and 1979, adenocarcinoma was found in 9.4%, and hyperplasias in 12.9% of the cases.[9] Nineteen of the 26 hyperplasias seen at Mount Sinai Medical Center were of the adenomatous type. Cystic glandular hyperplasia was found in 5 patients, and 2 patients had other hyperplastic changes, usually proliferative. Overall, 42% of the patients with postmenopausal bleeding studied at Mount Sinai Medical Center had been treated with estrogens; while 79% of the patients with adenomatous hyperplasia took these drugs, as mentioned above.

Seventeen per cent (39/233) of the endometrial curettings from women with postmenopausal bleeding evaluated at Mount Sinai Medical Center were classified as "non-phasic," because those endometrial samples were not characterized by the histologic features of proliferative endometrium, and they were not secretory. It has been suggested that the nonphasic pattern represents the effects of asynchronous hormonal stimulation. Of the postmenopausal patients without hyperplasia or carcinoma who received estrogens before uterine bleeding, 22% had nonphasic endometrium and 24% were found to have endometrial polyps. The endometrial curettings from 15% of these patients on estrogens were atrophic, but only 9% were classified as proliferative[9] (Table 2). On the other hand, 40-50% of patients gave a history of estrogen use whether their endometrial curettings showed atrophy, proliferation, polyps or were nonphasic. Obviously, there is no histologically typical endometrium which can be clearly associated with estrogen-stimulated postmenopausal bleeding; although so called "nonphasic" endometrium may

TABLE 2. ENDOMETRIAL HISTOLOGY IN PATIENTS WITH
POSTMENOPAUSAL UTERINE BLEEDING RELATED TO
EXOGENOUS ESTROGEN USE*
MOUNT SINAI MEDICAL CENTER, MILWAUKEE, 1975-1979[9]

	Total No. of Cases	Patients using estrogens	
		No.	(%)
Adenocarcinoma	22	6	(27)
Sarcoma	3	0	—
Hyperplasia			
Adenomatous	19	15	(79)
(Atypical/Adenomatous)	(5/19)	(4/5)	
Cystic glandular	5	1	(20)
Proliferative	2	1	(50)
Polyps	49	22	(45)
Nonphasic	39	20	(51)
Proliferative	17	8	(47)
Atrophic	32	14	(44)
Insufficient for diagnosis	24	5	(21)
Totals	212	92	(43)

*Overall, 98/233 patients with postmenopausal bleeding from all sites were using estrogens.

represent effects which can be ascribed only to long-term exposure to an unopposed estrogen milieu, whether endogenous or from exogenous medications.

Endometritis. Pyometrium or histologic evidence of nontuberculous endometritis will be found in a few patients with postmenopausal bleeding.[2,3,11] However, tuberculosis infection is now an extremely rare cause of endometrial bleeding in patients from Western countries.[4-11,41] Following menopause, stenosis of the uterine cervix by a neoplastic lesion may predispose to chronic endometritis. Because of the partial obstruction, incomplete evacuation of uterine contents leads to retention of debris and ultimately bacterial infection. Intermittent blood-tinged purulent discharge or the symptoms and signs of pelvic infection may be the harbinger of otherwise silent uterine tumors.

Although uterine myomata are frequent incidental findings, postmenopausal bleeding is rarely attributable to these benign tumors, even when they are in a submucosal position beneath the endometrium.[2,3,8,9,11,42] During the reproductive years, leiomyomata are frequent causes of symptomatic and asymptomatic uterine enlargement. It is important to emphasize that no growth should be experienced in these benign estrogen-dependent tumors following the cessation of regular cyclic ovarian hormonal stimulation at the time of menopause. Therefore, uterine growth or the *de novo* finding of an abnormal pelvic mass in a postmenopausal woman demands immediate steps to establish a diagnosis and rule out the presence of serious uterine or adnexal pathology.

Sarcomas. Postmenopausal bleeding is the most common presenting symptom of uterine sarcomas. While these uncommon malignant tumors were discovered as the cause of postmenopausal bleeding in only 1% of all patients reviewed,[2-4,8,9,11] it should be noted that sarcomas are relatively more often associated with postmenopausal bleeding than benign myomatous uterine tumors, which occur 100 times more frequently. When sarcomas are still confined to the uterine corpus, the prognosis is hopeful. However, bleeding may not be an early symptom in patients with uterine sarcomas, and very large tumors may first be evidenced only when they prolapse through the cervical canal accompanied by pain, bleeding and purulent discharge.

Uterine Tube: Fallopian tube cancers and inflammation are rare causes of postmenopausal bleeding (Table 1).[2,4,8-10] The uterine tube is the most unusual site of primary cancer in the female genital organs, but on the other hand, the highest incidence of tubal carcinoma does occur during the postmenopausal years. Complaints of pelvic pain and vaginal discharge should alert the practitioner to the possibility of this underlying disease. When first diagnosed, most tubal cancers have extended beyond the primary site, and in these patients the prognosis is extremely poor.[43]

Ovary: Although less than 5% of postmenopausal bleeding has been attributable to all forms of ovarian pathology, abnormal genital bleeding is one of the more common symptoms of ovarian cancer,[44,45] a disease of peak occurrence beyond the age of 40 years. Obviously, direct extension of ovarian cancer by invasion of the uterus and vagina may be manifest as postmenopausal bleeding, but the symptom of abnormal bleeding in the presence of ovarian neoplasms is probably as frequently the result of a more subtle mechanism. The continuous production of steroidal sex hormones by functional ovarian tumors provides uninterrupted estrogenic stimulation to the postmenopausal endometrium, sufficient to cause proliferation, hyperplasia and carcinoma.[44,45] Ovarian sex cord tumors of the granulosa-theca-lutein type have been associated with a 20% incidence of coexisting endometrial carcinoma in postmenopausal women.[44,46] However, benign and malignant ovarian cysts and tumors of epithelial origin are responsible for at least half of the postmenopausal bleeding caused by ovarian pathology.[45] There is accumulating data to support a concept that compression of ovarian stroma by enlarging primary cysts or masses, and even metastatic tumors to the ovaries, may induce the secretion of either or both estrogenic and androgenic hormones in amounts adequate to cause their usual end organ effects.[45,47-50] Screening methods for the detection of occult impalpable ovarian tumors, while still confined to the primary site, are poor; and signs or symptoms of early ovarian cancers are often lacking. Yet early diagnosis is crucial to achieving a favorable prognosis for patients with this dreadful disease. Prompt attention to the symptom of postmenopausal bleeding will undoubtedly uncover some malignant ovarian tumors that are still localized and amenable to control by surgical resection and appropriate adjuvant therapy.

Management of Postmenopausal Bleeding

The frequency with which malignant lesions are first evidenced by postmenopausal bleeding emphasizes the importance of an undelayed, judicious evaluation of all women with this symptom. Widespread acceptance of gynecologic screening has led to a considerable reduction in the incidence of invasive cervical carcinoma over the past 50 years. Furthermore, public education and undelayed institution of diagnostic measures also appear to be having an overall impact on lowering the proportion of patients with postmenopausal bleeding who are found to harbor cancerous tumors of any type.[2-9] These policies are to be encouraged. Still, during the past decade, there remains a 20-25% incidence of neoplastic and malignant disease in women who present with postmenopausal bleeding.[8,9]

Once established early in a woman's reproductive life, the individual cyclic menstrual pattern normally does not vary, except during times of pregnancy and lactation, until the perimenopausal years. At menopause, ovulation may cease abruptly. Other women may experience extended intervals of oligoovulation, sometimes lasting several months, during which menstruation does not occur—only then to resume again a normal cyclic withdrawal pattern. It is important to impress on the perimenopausal patient that although fertility may be diminished during this time, any ovulation provides the potential for conception. Any deviation from a woman's typical menstrual pattern demands attention and documentation. Unusual amounts or character of menses and extended, frequent or irregular menstrual flow should each be investigated in the perimenopausal female since heavy and/or irregular bleeding in this age group is associated with a significant incidence of pathology, including neoplasia.[51,52]

Postmenopausal bleeding, by convention, is any genital bleeding which occurs beyond twelve months after the last menstrual period at the menopause.[4] In any series, it is extremely difficult to document the occurrence of ovulation more than one year beyond the menopause. Secretory endometrium, as evidence of ovulation, was found on D&C in only 3 of 1,048 patients (0.3%) who were studied for postmenopausal bleeding.[2,4,9,11] Too often, advanced pelvic tumors are seen in postmenopausal women who have attributed their bleeding to "getting back my period." Only a single episode of postmenopausal bleeding was experienced by 15% of the patients found by Brewer and Miller to have gynecologic cancer.[4] It is unacceptable to dismiss without evaluation any woman who complains of genital bleeding which occurs more than one year following the menopause.

Outpatient Exam: The step-wise approach to evaluation of postmenopausal bleeding first entails a comprehensive personal and family history. All pertinent symptoms which are elicited must be investigated. Together with a complete general examination, a meticulous pelvic examination is performed during which particular attention is paid to the perineum and anus, vulva, introitus and peri-urethral areas, vagina and cervix. Bimanual palpation of the pelvic organs includes rectal examination and a test of any recovered feces for occult blood. All visible lesions are noted, and apparent genital age and evidence of mucosal estrogenization are correlated with chronologic age.

Pap smears. Cytologic smears of scrapings from the mid lateral vaginal sidewalls stained and examined with the Pap technique are often helpful in assessing the estrogen status by means of a relative maturation index. At Mount Sinai Medical Center, nine smears were available from postmenopausal patients who were not taking exogenous estrogens prior to being diagnosed as having endometrial neoplasms. Two of those smears showed squamous cell maturation consistent with increased endogenous estrogen production.[9] By the time of menopause, the squamocolumnar junction of the aging cervix has usually retracted to within the external os. Samples of the posterior vaginal pool, scrapings of the ectocervix and endocervical swab or aspiration should be done to screen the apparently normal postmenopausal cervix. Cytology obtained by directly scraping visible lesions may be helpful, and histologic diagnosis, frequently definitive, may be obtained through biopsy of lesions discovered during the initial examination.

Biopsies. A histologic diagnosis obtained early during the process of evaluation is often valuable in planning further tests and procedures prior to hospitalization. In the office or outpatient treatment room, small lesions of the perineum, vulva and vagina can often be excised *in toto* following infiltration with a local anesthetic agent. Larger lower genital lesions are frequently nonsensitive, and tiny representative pieces can usually be safely taken by incisional biopsy without the need for local anesthetic. Pigmented or apparently vascular lesions should be reserved for controlled excisional biopsies during hospitalization under anesthesia, usually with an experienced gynecologic oncologist in attendance or in consultation. Visible lesions of the upper vagina and cervix may be biopsied by means of a small sharp jawed forceps, such as the ones designed by Eppendorfer or Kevorkian.

Colposcopy. Colposcopic examination of the upper vagina and cervix may be helpful in delineating some lesions which could be misinterpreted by examination with the unaided eye. However, retraction of the squamocolumnar junction and thus the transitional zone into the endocervix during the perimenopausal years renders colposcopy less important than in the evaluation of cervical lesions and abnormal Pap smears during the earlier reproductive years.

As we consider the findings of the initial examination, it is important to note that the discovery of a cervical, lower genital tract or non-genital source of bleeding does not preclude the presence of another lesion higher in the uterus or adnexal organs. Cervical-vaginal Pap smears, while an important screening method for cervical neoplasia, are not reliable alone for the detection of endometrial cancer. Only 30-50% of endometrial cancers in several series were found to have suspicious or positive cervical-vaginal cytology.[31,35–39]

Endometrial screening. As a screening method, collection of fluids and tissues from within the uterine cavity for cytologic and histologic interpretation improves the yield in our efforts to detect occult endometrial cancer.[19,53,54] However, these procedures are not always sufficient to establish the cause of postmenopausal bleeding.[9,53,54] Such benign and premalignant pathology as polyps, myomas and hyperplasias may go undiagnosed and thereby untreated when these methods are used alone.[19,35,53] So while the addition of endometrial sampling to our armamentarium for screening asymptomatic postmenopausal women is laudatory, sole reliance upon these techniques to establish a tissue diagnosis and to rule out the possibility of neoplastic pathology is not sufficient in the face of frank postmenopausal bleeding.[35,54,55] Although there has been a movement by some investigators to carry out only outpatient endometrial sampling techniques, with or without endocervical curettage, in their evaluation of symptomatic patients,[56,57] the shortcomings of these methods and the importance of establishing the most reliable diagnosis possible in postmenopausal women with bleeding, leads me to recommend a thorough examination with anesthesia and fractional uterine curettage to complete the initial workup.[35]

In those cases in which invasive cancer has been detected during the outpatient evaluation, the involvement of a gynecologist with special expertise in oncology will often benefit the patient and her primary physician. Whenever practical, all first consultations should be obtained prior to making definite arrangements for hospital admission. Extraordinary findings of uterine size, shape or consistency, induration of the pelvic tissues and the presence of extrauterine masses will often dictate a need for further roentgenographic, scanning and endoscopic procedures, which may be scheduled before the hospitalization. Outpatient medical testing, effective communications between collaborating physicians, and careful planning of the hospital course are important to minimize the stay and lessen the economic impact.

Exam Under Anesthesia: The pivotal event in the evaluation of postmenopausal bleeding and the key to definitive diagnosis and further management is usually the examination under anesthesia and uterine curettage. These procedures may be accomplished with either general or regional anesthesia and should be done in an amply outfitted and supplied hospital operating room or adjacent outpatient surgical unit. Facilities for any untoward eventuality, including blood banking and full service laboratory and x-ray departments should be immediately available. Competent pathologic consultation with ability to perform and histologically interpret frozen tissue sections must also be at hand.

Inspection and palpation. Examination under anesthesia begins with the patient lying dorsally supine to permit thorough palpation of the abdomen and groins; she is then placed in a dorsal lithotomy position, unless anatomic abnormalities require some other suitable though compromised position. Following careful inspection and palpation of the vulva, perineum and introitus, including the urethra and areas of the Bartholin's and Skene's glands, the vagina is opened by firm but gentle digital pressure posteriorly against the perineal body. The vaginal mucosa is initially palpated, and a bivalve speculum of appropriate size and shape is progressively inserted under direct visualization until the cervix is fully exposed. At times, it may be necessary to use single blade retractors, such as those attributed to Sims, Heaney or Deaver, to permit this exposure. After careful inspection of the cervix, using a colposcope if indicated by the preadmission evaluation, the speculum is slowly withdrawn so that again the vaginal mucosa may be visualized. Bimanual vaginal and rectal-vaginal pelvic examinations are carried out with special attention to the submucosal tissues of the vagina and rectovaginal septum, bladder and urethra, paracervical tissues and uterosacral ligaments. The attitude, size, shape and consistency of the uterine cervix and corpus are noted, and the adnexae and posterior cul-de-sac are scrutinized. The nonfunctioning, atrophic senile ovary should not be enlarged and should no longer be palpable more than one or two years following menopause.[58,59] Therefore, the finding of any adnexal mass demands explanation.

The examination under anesthesia can be incredibly revealing. Intraperitoneal masses may be found which require further evaluation by noninvasive roentgenographic, radioisotope or ultrasound scanning techniques; or open inspection by laparoscopy or laparotomy may be necessary. Small lesions previously undisclosed during the preadmission examination may be discovered while the patient is under anesthesia and biopsied directly. Unsuspected induration and nodules may be considered for needle biopsy. Extreme caution should be exercised in undertaking the biopsy of pigmented lesions involving the vaginal or cervical mucosa. These may represent malignant melanomas or extensively infiltrating vascular tumors. When confronted with such lesions, no matter how small, consultation with a gynecologic oncologist is wise.

Abnormal Pap smears. Cytologic smears, unexplained by or inconsistent with preliminary biopsies obtained during the preadmission workup, should not be dismissed without establishing an accurate histologic diagnosis. With the patient under general anesthesia, a searching reexamination of the lower genital tract and cervix, both visually and by means of colposcopy, may disclose previously unnoticed lesions and mucosal patterns to be approached by directed biopsies. When small, early epithelial neoplasms of the vagina or cervix have been diagnosed during the preadmission workup, they may adequately and appropriately be treated by local excision at these times. More widespread but early intraepithelial neoplasms may be destroyed by carefully directed cautery, cryosurgery or laser therapy. Severe intraepithelial lesions and those with early stromal invasion on preliminary biopsies must be further defined by complete excision designed to include a surrounding margin of normal mucosa and underlying stroma. When such severe lesions arise on the cervix, or cervical intraepithelial neoplasia (CIN) of *any* degree extends beyond view into the endocervical canal, complete excision can usually be most effectively accomplished by surgical conization of the cervix designed to encompass the entire transitional zone and all abnormal areas as defined by colposcopy and Lugol's iodine staining. Conization is followed by small four quadrant punch biopsies taken from the endocervical canal above the apex of the cone by means of a laryngeal forceps and then curettage at the level of the internal os.

Such a careful, systematic approach, which costs little in time or energy, may disclose the presence of neoplastic disease beyond the extent of the cervical cone, especially in postmenopausal women where the squamocolumnar junction has often ascended high into the cervical canal.[60] Squamous cell dysplasia, and even invasive cancer, may involve deeply penetrating endocervical glands at this level. Furthermore, the not infrequent coexistence of adenocarcinoma *in situ* with squamous dysplasia should be noted, since foci of adenocarcinoma *in situ* have been found in cervical tissues of the upper canal when lower and more superficial glands were normal.[9,60]

Cervical conization should *not* be carried out when a definitive diagnosis of invasive cancer can be achieved through punch biopsies. Cone biopsy of a cervix containing invasive carcinoma is associated with a significant incidence of parametritis and frequent severe hemorrhagic complications, which may compromise subsequent oncologic management. The operating room examination under anesthesia offers an opportunity to obtain biopsies which may be difficult to accomplish on the unanesthetized elderly patient in a treatment room setting. When the physical findings have raised the suspicion of invasive cancer, but this diagnosis is not corroborated by the histology seen on preliminary biopsies, additional tissues should be obtained by means of punch or needle biopsies before proceeding to conization. Frozen section examination of these tissues will often be diagnostic, but where it is not and suspicion of invasion runs high, it may be prudent to obtain additional biopsies and/or await the study of permanent sections, delaying the conization for a later date, in case this procedure may be avoided.

Uterine Curettage: In virtually every case of postmenopausal bleeding which has not been previously evaluated, a fractional uterine curettage (D&C) is indicated to complete the diagnostic workup. This is true even when a lower tract lesion, cervical disease, prolapsed endometrial polyp or adnexal pathology are discovered. For, as we have seen, none of these entities will preclude the coexistence of additional intrauterine pathology. When cervical conization is done as described above, it is always carried out prior to D&C, so as not to disrupt the endocervical glands and stroma, proper orientation of which are so vital to histopathologic diagnosis. Similarly, when conization is not done, uterine sounding and dilation of the internal os are always reserved until after completion of the endocervical curettage.

Proper, orderly performance of the fractional D&C is essential for accurate interpretation of the operative findings and recovered tissues. Following bimanual examination with delineation of uterine size and attitude, the cervix is exposed and grasped through the portio vaginalis with one or two fine single tooth tenaculae. Before the uterus is sounded or the cervix is dilated, previously unsampled cervical lesions, if present, should be biopsied. Then using a small sharp curette, such as the one designed by Kevorkian and Younge, curettage of the full extent of the endocervix is carried out with special care not to proceed beyond the internal os. A thorough deep endocervical curettage is accomplished by exerting sufficient pressure to disengage endocervical mucosa and some underlying stroma. Often four quadrant swipes followed by circumferential scraping of the entire endocervix is useful in accomplishing this.

When adenocarcinoma is discovered in endocervical curettings, it is vitally important to future management that the operator be assured that these tissues have been obtained directly from the cervical canal. Only after completion of the endocervical curettage is the uterine cavity sounded, measured and assessed for volume and deviation. At times, the postmenopausal cervix is so firm and constricted that it is not possible to readily pass a standard uterine sound. For these cases, the surgeon should be equipped with a fine malleable probe, which can usually be passed to "pave the way" for probes and sounds of larger caliber. By using these techniques when needed, one is able to probe the cervix and sound the cavity in most patients who have demonstrated postmenopausal uterine bleeding.

When purulent material is encountered, a small syringe with a flexible 14 gauge cannula should be available to withdraw fluid directly from the uterus for aerobic and anaerobic cultures. Culture swabs also may be passed into the uterus and immediately placed in a carrying medium to complete the bacteriologic sampling. Care must be taken not to break a wooden culture stick within the uterus, and therefore plastic swabs are preferred. If granulomatous infection is suspected, endometrial tissues recovered by curettage can be taken for special cultures and stains.

Gentle and progressive dilation of the endocervix is accomplished by means of graduated instruments of the Hegar or Hank variety. My own preference often is to use graduated Delclos dilators, which are deeply scored at standard intervals, enabling accurate measurement of the uterine depth, and curved so as to permit angulation and passage of these instruments into uteri where this achievement may be more difficult with probes and sounds of straighter design. The internal os is dilated just enough to allow free and easy passage of small to medium-size malleable endometrial curettes. Bending the curette, as is necessary to follow the curve of the uterine cavity, systematic sharp curettage of the endometrium is carried out with special attention to swipe across the fundus and explore the cornuae. To avoid inadvertent injury, care and diligence must be exercised during curettage of the often small, distorted and fragile postmenopausal uterus. When it is clear to the gynecologic surgeon that thorough endometrial curettage has been accomplished and little if any tissues are recovered, the temptation to "dig more deeply" should be resisted. Recovered tissues are continuously monitored by gross inspection and histologic study of suspicious material.

Once a diagnosis of frankly invasive cancer in the uterine curettings can be made, it is usually unnecessary and frequently undesirable to continue the procedure of sharp curettage. Too often, overzealous curettage by inexperienced operators has led to serious hemorrhage and dangerous perforations. Complications of bleeding, peritoneal infection, dissemination of neoplastic disease, injury to intra-abdominal viscera and the necessary compromises of therapy which must follow uterine perforations, may cost the patient her very life. In the case of suspected uterine perforation, the procedure should cease immediately, and the perforation ascertained by gentle probing when possible, because such an injury may have bearing on later decisions regarding intracavitary radiotherapy if cancer is discovered.

Upon completion of the endometrial curettage, curved common duct forceps or some similar instrument is introduced to search for polyps which may not have been dislodged by the sharp curette and would otherwise escape detection.[34] These polyp forceps are opened and closed several times against each sidewall and fundus of the uterine cavity and withdrawn with each manipulation. Finally, a small to medium-size smooth curette is employed to explore the entire endometrial surface for any irregularities. When present, such surface irregularities usually represent submucosal uterine leiomyomata. However, these benign tumors are only a rare cause of uterine bleeding after menopause.[2-9,42] When postmenopausal bleeding is associated with this finding, the physician should be alert to the need for followup at planned intervals with pelvic examinations and documentation of uterine size by palpation and possibly with scanning techniques in order to assure the impression of benign leiomyomata and minimize the possibility of missing more serious intramural tumors.

Nondefinitive Findings: Approximately one in ten (24/233) of the women evaluated for postmenopausal bleeding at our Medical Center between 1975 and 1979 were discharged without a definitive histologic diagnosis or a defined cause of bleeding.[9] Nine of these 24 patients had undergone previous nondefinitive workup for abnormal bleeding. However, recurrent bleeding can not be disregarded. Of 51 uterine cancers and hyperplasias discovered in this series, 18 had previously been evaluated for abnormal bleeding. These included 5 invasive endometrial carcinomas, 8 adenomatous or atypical endometrial hyperplasias and 1 sarcoma. Thus, 19% of the 73 women evaluated for recurrent postmenopausal bleeding in this series were found to have uterine cancers or premalignant hyperplasias.[9] Eleven of the 13 recurrent bleeders with endometrial cancers or adenomatous hyperplasias were taking exogenous estrogens (85%); while 49% (30/61) of all other women with recurrent bleeding had received these drugs. This is not a significant difference from the 42% use of exogenous estrogens in the overall series of postmenopausal bleeders evaluated at Mount Sinai Medical Center.[9] We may speculate that, whether or not exogenous estrogens played a role in the development of neoplastic endometrial lesions, the use of these medications may have served to unmask serious pathology which had gone unnoticed at the time of prior examinations.

A generation ago, Brewer and Miller advocated the use of prophylactic hysterectomy in patients with postmenopausal bleeding for whom a definitive diagnosis could not be established.[4] As noted then by TeLind,[61] this aggressive approach was difficult to justify even at that time, especially in view of the predominantly benign lesions in the remainder of Brewer and Miller's patients.[4,61] With the accumulation of further data and the availability of revealing screening measures, such a recommendation for major surgery must be considered radical today. Over 80% of the recurrent postmenopausal bleeding evaluated at Mount Sinai Medical Center, Milwaukee, was due to benign conditions.[9] On the other hand, as noted above, 14 neoplastic lesions, including 6 invasive cancers, were discovered in the Mount Sinai series through examination under anesthesia and D&C of 73 postmenopausal women who had been previously evaluated for abnormal bleeding. The practitioner is bound to do all that is possible to ascertain the absence of neoplastic disease or adequately treat that which may be present. Therefore, it behooves those caring for postmenopausal women to undertake a careful plan of followup by physical examination and screening and scanning techniques in any case in which the symptom of uterine bleeding cannot be fully explained by the findings on initial evaluation. In older patients, special efforts must be invoked to insure that no woman under such a regimen of management is lost to medical attention. Fortunately, heretofore social resources have been intact to assist the physician in this task.

Follow Up

In the course of following women who have demonstrated postmenopausal bleeding in the absence of exogenous estrogens, there may be merit in the "progestogen challenge test," as advanced by Gambrell et al.[62] Data presented by those authors show a lower rate of endometrial carcinomas among estrogen-treated patients who have been given superimposed progestogens during the last 10 days of each monthly cycle than was found either in those women treated with estrogens alone or in the untreated population attending their clinics in Texas.[29,62] That approach to the use of therapeutic hormones is advocated by Gambrell and his coworkers for those menopausal women who would be expected to benefit from estrogen replacement therapy.[29] Cyclic buildup and shedding of endometrium primed by endogenous estrogens through the administration of progestogen for the last 10 days of each month might also be prophylactic in preventing endometrial hyperplasia and carcinoma.[62,63]

In a series of postmenopausal patients diagnosed with endometrial carcinoma at New Britain General Hospital, Connecticut, between 1971 and 1977, only 32.9% had abnormal cervical-vaginal Pap smears,[31] and only 7.8% of endometrial cancers occurring in postmenopausal women of an earlier series from that hospital were diagnosed as the result of cervical-vaginal cytologic screening of asymptomatic patients.[35] Pap smears were available on 10 of the 14 patients with cancers and premalignant hyperplasias in the recurrent bleeding group evaluated at our medical center, but only one of these showed abnormal endometrial cells.[9] Six of the 11 Pap smears available for review from postmenopausal bleeders with endometrial cancers were suspicious or positive; however, none of the available Pap smears from patients with adenomatous hyperplasia was read as abnormal.[9] Nevertheless, cervical-vaginal Pap smears do detect endometrial pathology in some women,[31,35-37] and this method is of great value in screening for cervical neoplasia, which may also present in the postmenopausal female. The presence of even normal endometrial cells in the Pap smears of postmenopausal women should be regarded as suspicious for endometrial pathology. Ng et al. found a 5.7% incidence of endometrial cancer and a 13.2% incidence of hyperplasia in postmenopausal women with normal endometrial cells in their Pap smears.[64] This test is simple, painless and relatively inexpensive and should not be abandoned in the postmenopausal woman.

Endometrial sampling techniques are accurate in the detection of frankly invasive carcinoma, and are important adjuncts to physical examination and cervical-vaginal Pap smears in screening for this disease in asymptomatic women.[19,53,54] These methods should certainly be invoked in the followup of patients who have experienced menometrorrhagia in the perimenopausal years and in all who have had postmenopausal uterine bleeding. For, as we have noted, a substantial number of these women may harbor or subsequently develop a malignant neoplasm. Furthermore, in the Mount Sinai Medical Center series, a relatively high proportion of these women (59%) either have been treated with estrogenic medications or have evidence of endogenous estrogenization, both associated with a predilection for endometrial hyperplasia and carcinoma.[9]

All cytohistologic screening of postmenopausal patients should begin with an aspiration from the endocervix and a direct scraping of the entire transitional zone, which has usually retracted into the endocervix by the time of menopause.[19] Samples of the posterior vaginal pool may yield otherwise undetected endometrial cells.[54] Vaginal sidewall scrapings are obtained for evaluation of the estrogen status by a maturation index of the squamous cells. Material satisfactory for cytologic evaluation is recovered directly from the endometrial cavity by uterine aspiration and lavage techniques.[53,54] The Gravlee jet endometrial washer also recovers dislodged tissues which are suitable for histologic evaluation.[53] Biopsy devices and suction curettes provide endometrial tissues which may be more readily processed and interpreted in clinical laboratories that are not specially devoted to cytologic preparation and diagnosis of materials recovered by endometrial irrigation.

Postmenopausal bleeding is a symptom which still heralds a significant amount of serious pathology. At least 20-30% of women with this symptom are found to have malignant or premalignant neoplasms. These generally arise in the endometrium, but other uterine corpus, cervical, ovarian and lower tract lesions, as well as tumors of the bowel and urinary system may be responsible. The development of endometrial hyperplasias and carcinomas is associated with unopposed endogenous estrogen secretion and exogenous estrogen administration. Systematic evaluation of all cases of postmenopausal bleeding is required. Patients with postmenopausal bleeding in whom definitive surgical therapy is not indicated, must be followed throughout life with a planned course of interval reevaluation, including physical examination, cytohistologic studies and scanning techniques in selected cases.

REFERENCES

1. Payne, F.S.: Causes of abnormal vaginal bleeding during the pre and postmenopausal ages. Med. Clin. N. Am. 20: 83-92, 1936.
2. Taylor, H.C., Jr. and Millen, R.: Causes of vaginal bleeding and the history of the endometrium after the menopause. Am. J. Obstet. Gynecol. 36:22-39, 1938.
3. Jones, B.D., Jr., and Cantor, E.B.: Postmenopausal bleeding and its management. A ten-year survey. Am. J. Obstet. Gynecol. 62:365-369, 1951.
4. Brewer, J.L. and Miller, W.H.: Postmenopausal uterine bleeding. Am. J. Obstet. Gynecol. 67:988-1013, 1954.
5. Woodruff, J.D., Prystowsky, H. and TeLinde, R.W.: Postmenopausal bleeding. A re-evaluation of an old problem. S. Med. J. 51:302-305,1958.
6. Payne, F.L., Wright, R.C. and Fetterman, H.H.: Postmenopausal bleeding. Am. J. Obstet. Gynecol. 77:1216-1227, 1959.
7. Collins, C.G. and Jansen, F.W.: Menopausal and postmenopausal bleeding. J. Arkansas Med. Soc. 56:429-434, 1960.
8. Hawwa, Z.M., Nahhas, W.A. and Copenhaver, E.H.: Postmenopausal bleeding. Lahey Clin. Found. Bull. 19:61-70, 1970.
9. Casey, M.J.: Mount Sinai Medical Center, Milwaukee, Wisc., unpublished data, 1982.
10. Israel, S.L. and Weber, L.L.: Postmenopausal uterine bleeding. Obstet. Gynecol. 7:286-292, 1956.
11. Brzezinsky, A. and Bromberg, Y.M.: Significance of postmenopausal genital bleeding in Jewish women. Obstet. Gynecol. 1:359-363, 1953.
12. Mikail, G.: Sex steroids in blood. Clin. Obstet. Gynecol. 10:29-39, 1967.
13. MacDonald, P.C., Rombault, R.P. and Siiteri, P.K.: Plasma precursors of estrogen. I. Extent of conversion of plasma Δ - androstenedione to estrone in normal males and nonpregnant, normal, castrate and adrenalectomized females. J. Clin. Endocrin. 27:1103-1111, 1967.
14. Gambrell, R.D., Jr.: Postmenopausal bleeding. J. Am. Ger. Soc. 22:337-343, 1974.
15. Greenblatt, R.B., Dettinger, M. and Bohler, C. S-S.: Estrogen-androgen levels in aging men and women: Therapeutic considerations. J. Am. Ger. Soc. 24:173-178, 1976.
16. Greenblatt, R.B., Colle, M.L. and Mahesh, V.B.: Ovarian and adrenal steroid production in the postmenopausal woman. Obstet. Gynecol. 7:383-387, 1976.
17. Schindler, A.E., Ebert, A. and Friedrich, E.: Conversion of androstenedione to estrone by human fat tissue. J. Clin. Endocrin., Metab. 35:627-630, 1972
18. MacDonald, P.C., Edman, C.D., Hemsell, D.L., Porter, J.C. and Siiteri, P.K.: Effect of obesity on conversion of plasma androstenedione to estrone in postmenopausal women with and without endometrial cancer. Am. J. Obstet. Gynecol. 130:448-455, 1978.
19. Casey, M.J.: Estrogens, menopause and cancer. Conn. Med. 41:776-791, 1977.

20. Marshall, D.H., Fearnley, M., Holmes, A. and Nordin, B.E.C.: Relation between androstenedione and estrone levels in peri- and postmenopausal women in *Consensus on Menopausal Research,* van Keep, P.A., Greenblatt, R.B. and Albeaux-Fernet, M. (eds.) Lancaster, MTP Press Limited, 1976, pp. 100-108.

21. Gusberg, S.B.: Individual at high risk for endometrial carcinoma. Am. J. Obstet. Gynecol. 126:535-542, 1976.

22. Wortsman, J., Singh, K.B., and Murphy, J.: Evidence for the hypothalamic origin of the polycystic ovary syndrome. Obstet. Gynecol. 58:137-141, 1981.

23. Dockerty, M.B., Lovelady, S.B. and Foust, G.T., Jr.: Carinoma of the corpus uteri in young women. Am. J. Obstet. Gynecol. 61:966-981, 1951.

24. Dockerty, M.B. and Mussey, E.: Malignant lesions of the uterus associated with estrogen producing ovarian tumors. Am. J. Obstet. Gynecol. 61:147-153, 1951.

25. Cutler, B.S., Forbes, A.P., Ingersoll, F.M. and Scully, R.E.: Endometrial carcinoma after stilbestrol therapy in gonadal dysgenesis. N. Eng. J. Med. 287:628-631, 1972.

26. Lyon, F.A.: Development of adenocarcinoma of the endometrium in young women receiving long-term sequential oral contraceptives. Am. J. Obstet. Gynecol. 123:299-301, 1975.

27. Smith, D.C., Prentice, R., Thompson, D.J. and Herrmann, W.L.: Association of exogenous estrogen and endometrial carcinoma. N. Eng. J. Med. 293: 1164-1167, 1975.

28. Ziel, H.K. and Finkle, W.D.: Increased risk of endometrial carcinoma among users of conjugated estrogens. N. Eng. J. Med. 293:1167-1170, 1975.

29. Gambrell, R.D., Massey, F.M., Castaneda, T.A., Ugenas, A.J., Ricci, C.A.: Reduced incidence of endometrial cancer among postmenopausal women treated with progestogens. J. Am. Ger. Soc. 27:389-394, 1979.

30. Kistner, R.W.: Effects of progestational agents on hyperplasia and carcinoma *in situ* of the endometrium, in *Gynecologic Oncology. A Comprehensive Review and Evaluation,* Barber, H.R.K. and Graber, E.A. (eds.) Baltimore, The Williams & Wilkins Company, 1970, pp. 141-155.

31. Kennedy, A.W., Casey, M.J., Gondos, B. and McLucas, E.G.H.: Carcinoma of the endometrium: Review of experience at a community hospital, 1971-1977. Gynecol. Oncol. 14:164-174, 1982.

32. Chung, A.F., Woodruff, J.M. and Lewis, J.L., Jr.: Malignant melanoma of the vulva: A report of 44 cases. Obstet. Gynecol. 45:638-646, 1975.

33. Chung, A.F., Casey, M.J., Flannery, J.T., Woodruff, J.M. and Lewis. J.L., Jr.: Malignant melanomas of the vagina - Report of 19 cases. Obstet. Gynecol. 55:720-727, 1980.

34. Peterson, W.F. and Novak, E.R.: Endometrial polyps. Obstet. Gynecol. 8:40-49, 1956.

35. Casey, M.J., Madden, T.J., McLucas, E. and Kennedy, A.W.: Endometrium in the postmenopause, presented at the Second International Congress on the Menopause, Jerusalem, June 4-9, 1978.

36. Nahhas, W.A., Lund, C.J. and Rudolph, J.H.: Carcinoma of the corpus

uteri. A 10-year review of 225 patients. Obstet. Gynecol. 38:564-570, 1971.
37. Jones, W.E., Kanner, H.M., Kanner, H.H. and Benson, C.: Adenocarcinoma of the endometrium: Twenty-five years' experience in private practice. Am. J. Obstet. Gynecol. 113:549-557, 1972.
38. Frick, H.C., II, Munnel, E.W., Richart, R.M., Berger, A.P. and Lawry, M.F.: Carcinoma of the endometrium. Am. J. Obstet. Gynecol. 115: 663-676. 1973.
39. Jones, H.W., III: Treatment of adenocarcinoma of the endometrium. Obstet. Gynecol. Sur. 30:147-169, 1975.
40. Homesley, H.D., Boronow, R.C. and Lewis, J.L., Jr.: Treatment of carcinoma of the endometrium at Memorial-James Ewing Hospital, 1949-1965. Obstet. Gynecol. 47:100-105, 1976.
41. Sutherland, A.M.: Genital tuberculosis in women. Am. J. Obstet. Gynecol. 79:486-497, 1960.
42. Duckman, S., Sese, L., Suarez, J. and Tantakesem, P.: Myoma uteri and abnormal uterine bleeding. S. Med. J. 65:1356-1359, 1972.
43. Boutselis, J.G. and Thompson, J.N.: Clinical aspects of primary carcinoma of the fallopian tube. A clinical study of 14 cases. Am. J. Obstet. Gynecol. 111:98-101, 1981.
44. Dockerty, M.B. and Mussey, E.: Malignant lesions of the uterus associated with estrogen producing ovarian tumors. Am. J. Obstet. Gynecol. 61:147-153, 1961.
45. Rome, R.M., Laverty, C.R., and Brown, J.B.: Ovarian tumors in postmenopausal women. J. Obstet. Gynecol. Brit. Common. 80:984-991, 1973.
46. Hertig, A.T.: Endocrine ovarian-cancer relationships. Cancer 10:838-841, 1957.
47. Scott J.S., Lumsdam, C.E. and Levell, M.J.: Ovarian endocrine activity in association with hormonally inactive neoplasia. Am. J. Obstet. Gynecol. 97:161-170, 1967.
48. MacDonald, P.C., Grodin, J.M., Edman, C.D., Vellios, F. and Siiteri, P.K.: Origin of estrogen in a postmenopausal women with a nonendocrine tumor of the ovary and endometrial hyperplasia. Obstet. Gynecol. 47:644-650, 1976.
49. Turunen, A.: Hormonal secretion of Krukenberg tumors. Acta Endocrinol. 20:50-56, 1955.
50. Ober, W.B., Pollak, A., Gerstmann, K.E., and Kupperman, H.S.: Krukenberg tumor with androgenic and progestational activity. Am. J. Obstet. Gynecol. 84:739-744, 1962.
51. Millen, R.S. and Shepard, K.: Association of vaginal bleeding to organic pathology and the endometrial pattern in the decades before the menopause. Am. J. Obstet. Gynecol. 45:812-821, 1943.
52. Randall, C.L.: Recognition and management of the women predisposed to uterine adenocarcinoma. JAMA 127:20-25, 1945.
53. Casey, M.J. and Madden, T.J.: Experience with endometrial irrigations in menopausal women, in Consenus on Menopausal Research, van Keep, P.A., Greenblatt, R.B. and Albeaux-Fernet, M. (eds.), Lancaster, MTP Press Limited, 1976, pp. 139-151.

54. Kawada, C.Y. and An-Foraker, S.H.: Screening for endometrial carcinomas. Clin. Obstet. Gynecol. 22:713-728, 1979.
55. Anderson, D.G., Eaton, C.J., Galinkin, L.J., Newton, C.W., III, Haines, J.P. and Miller, N.F.: Cytologic diagnosis of endometrial adenocarcinoma. Am. J. Obstet. Gynecol. 125:376-383, 1976.
56. Underwood, P.B., Kellett, M.P., McKee,, E.E., and Clark, A.: Gravlee Jet Washer: Can it replace the diagnostic curettage? Am. J. Obstet. Gynecol 117:201-209, 1973.
57. Delke, I., Veridiano, N.P. and Diamond, B.: Vabra aspiration in office gynecology. Gynecol. Oncol. 10:329-336, 1980.
58. Barber, H.R.K. and Graber, E.A.: The PMPO syndrome (postmenopausal palpable ovary syndrome). Obstet. Gynecol. 38:921-923, 1971.
59. Barber, H.R.K.: *Ovarian Cancer. Etiology, Diagnosis and Treatment,* New York, Masson Publishing USA, Inc., 1978, pp. 175-178.
60. Weisbrot, I.W., Stabinsky, C. and Davis, A.M.: Adenocarcinoma *in situ* of the uterine cervix. Cancer 29:1179-1187, 1972.
61. TeLind, R.: Discussion. Postmenopausal bleeding. Am. J. Obstet Gynecol. 67:1011, 1954.
62. Gambrell, R.D., Massey, F.M., Castaneda, T.A., Ugenas, A.J., Ricci, C.A. and Wright, J.M.: Use of the progestogen challenge test to reduce the risk of endometrial cancer. Obstet. Gynecol. 55:732-738, 1980.
63. Sturdee, D.W., Wade-Evans, T., Paterson, M.E.L., Thom, M. and Studd, J.W.W.: Relations between bleeding pattern, endometrial histology and estrogen therapy in menopausal women. Brit. Med. J. 1:1575-1577, 1978.
64. Ng, A.B.P., Reagan, J.W., Hawliczek, S. and Wentz, B.W.: Significance of endometrial cells in the detection of endometrial carcinoma and its precursors. Acta Cytol. 18:356-361, 1974.

8

URETHROVESICAL PROBLEMS IN FEMALE GERIATRIC PATIENTS

C. PAUL HODGKINSON, M.D.

The major urethrovesical problems in the aging female are those of urinary control, physiologic regressive changes incidental to estrogen deficiency, and anatomic derangements incidental to uterovaginal prolapse. Although none of these conditions qualifies specifically as a geriatric disease, they do frequently complicate the aging process of women 70 years of age or older. As was noted in the chapter on carcinoma of the breast, there is no specific age limit implied by the definition of geriatrics; however, for this project it is necessary to be arbitrary. Elderly is defined as that time of life when one is approaching average life expectancy, which in women is between 70 and 72 years. Because many women live much longer, geriatrics is defined as life beyond 72 years. It has been convenient to further divide this group into the "young" geriatric group, between 70 and 80 years old, and the "old" geriatric group, beyond 80 years. At age 80, there is necessarily considerable overlap, particularly for women, because some women are in considerably better health than others.

The Bladder and Old Age

Recently Hodgkinson, Dirghangi, and Salako reported a study of physiologic bladder capacity and residual urine values in 303 adult women with normal detrusor function.[1] Definite changes were noted in the 43 women aged 70 years and older. The study patients were divided into 2 groups: 124 who had no stress urinary incontinence (No SUI) and 179 who had clinical stress urinary incontinence (SUI). The overall mean bladder capacity for the entire group of 303 patients was 567 ml. For the No SUI group of 124, the mean was 488 ml, and for the 179 in the SUI group, 624 ml. The difference in the means for the 2 groups was 135 ml, with a significant p value of > 0.0005.

When the 43 patients 70 years old and older were analyzed separately, it was found that the mean bladder capacity was only 448 ml—a difference of 119 ml from the mean of the total 303 patients. Similarly, for the No SUI group, the mean was 410 ml, and for the SUI group, 484—a difference of 78 ml and 140 ml, respectively, from the 303. In the patients 70 years of age or older, the difference in the means was only 73 ml. Thus, after the age of 70, the overall bladder capacity tended to be reduced compared to the younger age group, and the differential between the No SUI group and SUI group was reduced to an insignificant figure.

The residual urine value for the 43 patients 70 years and older was 52 ml compared to 68 ml for the entire group of 303 patients. The difference of 16 ml was not considered significant except to indicate that patients over the age of 70 voided as well as the younger patients.

Difficulties in Urinary Control in the Aging Female

Urinary incontinence in the aging female can usually be identified as that due to detrusor dysfunction or that due to anatomic stress urinary incontinence. At that age there is also a small percentage of patients whose incontinence has persisted after repeated failed operative procedures for stress urinary incontinence.

In those with urinary incontinence due to detrusor dysfunction (identified as detrusor dyssynergia by direct electronic urethrocystometry), the etiology may be idiopathic or neurogenic. In many cases detrusor dysfunction develops as the result of neurogenic changes incidental to diabetes mellitus, spinal osteoporosis, or osteoarthritis. Definitive treatment is usually difficult. Early in their involvement, patients may respond to anticholinergic drugs, but with advancing disease drugs are frequently of no avail. Such anticholinergic drugs as Ditropan and Ornade Spansules may be contraindicated in the aging female because of conditions such as narrow-angle glaucoma, arterial hypertension, diabetes mellitus, dizziness, mental confusion, intestinal atony, and fecal impaction. Unfortunately, because of arterial hypertension many geriatric patients are receiving drug therapy that promotes diuresis. The increased urine output causes aggravation of the incontinence. If possible, quick-acting, short-term diuretics should be used rather than long-acting drugs so that the diuresis occurs during the day rather than at night. In cases of idiopathic detrusor dysfunction, drugs may or may not be effectual. Fortunately, this type of incontinence occurs infrequently. Treatment consists of control of urinary infection and perineal padding for the control of almost constant drainage of urine. Strict attention must be given to personal hygiene. Transurethral catheter drainage may be used temporarily, but this usually leads to aggravation of infection. Fortunately, more efficient perineal padding has recently become commercially available, e.g., Depend Undergarments (Kimberly-Clark Corporation, Neenah, Wisconsin).

Persistent urinary incontinence following multiple failed gynecologic operations for stress urinary incontinence is usually on an anatomic basis. This distressing condition is usually refractory to any form of treatment. Such patients generally have bladders with very small capacity and are plagued by frequent recurrent bladder infections. Treatment is most unsatisfactory and is similar to that for recalcitrant detrusor dysfunction.

Another anatomic type of incontinence frequently seen in the aged is stress urinary incontinence. Age per se is not a contraindication to appropriate surgery for pure anatomic stress urinary incontinence provided the diagnosis is accurately established without question. Detrusor dysfunction combined with anatomic stress urinary incontinence occurs with increased frequency in the geriatric patient. Operations for stress urinary incontinence do not correct detrusor dysfunction, and if the detrusor dyssynergia is not corrected, the patient is no better from a symptomatic standpoint. It is hazardous to perform a stress incontinence operation in a patient over 70 on the basis of history and physical examination alone. Preoperative comprehensive urodynamic investigation is a must for patients in this category.

Iatrogenic factors may adversely influence the tolerance of the patient over 70 years of age to operation. Many geriatric patients are undergoing treatment for systemic disease. The systemic effects of drug therapy for arterial hypertension, cardiac disease, diabetes mellitus, asthma, emphysema, or chronic respiratory disease must be carefully evaluated. Thiazide therapy and its effects on electrolytes needs to be investigated preoperatively. A careful history is imperative. Rauwolfia compounds, adrenocorticosteroids, anticoagulative preparations, opiates, barbiturates, and belladonna-like drugs are but a few that may increase the risk of surgery. It is important to remember that the older patient can usually withstand the operative procedure without difficulty, but she may have great difficulty withstanding the complications. Surgical technique must be meticulous. However, given a diagnosis of pure anatomic stress urinary incontinence in the absence of severe limiting health disabilities, retropubic urethropexy operative procedures are usually well tolerated and very successful. The oldest patient on whom I have operated for pure stress urinary incontinence was 84 years of age. She was most grateful for her complete relief of incontinence and lived a comfortable life for an additional 5 years. The significance of urinary incontinence in the geriatric patient population cannot be overestimated. The supervisor of a Presbyterian Home recently advised me that urinary incontinence was a problem for about one-third of the aged female residents.

Physiologic Changes Incidental to Estrogen Deficiency

Estrogen-regressive changes incidental to estrogen deficiency affect all geriatric patients to some degree. Most of the atrophic changes associated with estrogen deficiency directly affect the vagina and labia. Vaginal atrophy, vaginal stenosis, dyspareunia, labial adhesions, and uterovaginal prolapse are observed commonly in geriatric patients.

However, the lower urinary tract may be secondarily involved. As the result of senile vaginal atrophy, the support to the urethra is altered and the urethral mucosa shares in the atrophy. The mucosa of the external urethral meatus becomes exposed, making it more susceptible to trauma and infection. Urethral caruncles are commonly observed in the elderly female, and they may cause infection and severe pain. Treatment consists of excision of the caruncle.

In aged debilitated females, especially those with the increased chronic expiratory pressure that occurs in chronic asthma, chronic coughing, straining at stool, and crying, the entire urethral mucosa may prolapse through the external urinary meatus and thus cause swelling, strangulation, and gangrene. This condition is also seen in infants as a result of crying. Treatment consists of passing a catheter into the bladder and amputating the prolapsed mucosa. The healthy mucosal edges must be approximated by fine suturing.

Rarely, labial adhesions completely obstruct the vaginal introitus except for a tiny opening through which urine is expelled. This results in chronic urinary obstruction of the lower urinary tract. The labial adhesions can be separated manually with the patient under anesthesia. To prevent recurrence, estrogen creams or systemic estrogen therapy must be consistently employed. Mild stress urinary incontinence may occur as a result of estrogen deficiency. Response to adequate estrogen therapy may be very effective.

In all of these conditions, estrogen therapy is both prophylactic and curative. Most of the local conditions respond best to estrogen vaginal creams. Unfortunately, vaginal hygiene in the aged female is frequently neglected, as is gynecologic examination unless there is persistent bleeding. Even vaginal bleeding is often overlooked because of poor eyesight. Attendants should be warned to report blood stains on undergarments, on bed clothing, and in toilet bowls.

Varying degrees of uterovaginal prolapse are common problems of the aged female. Milder forms in the sedentary aged female may require no treatment, but extensive uterovaginal prolapse may result in vaginal ulceration, bleeding, and discharge. If extreme, uterovaginal prolapse may prevent voiding and cause urinary obstruction. Many patients with this difficulty learn to replace the prolapse into the vagina when attempting to void.

The ideal treatment for uterovaginal prolapse at any age is vaginal hysterectomy and anterior-posterior colporrhaphy. In an occasional geriatric patient, however, general health problems may be so precarious as to contraindicate anesthesia by Le Fort colpocleisis. However, this procedure is frequently followed by the development of severe stress urinary incontinence. Surgical correction of stress urinary incontinence following Le Fort operation is complicated and difficult.

In an occasional patient in whom no surgical procedure can be undertaken without extreme risk, a vaginal pessary may be used to support the prolapse. Although the use of a pessary is considerably less than ideal treatment, its use is at times necessary. When a pessary is inserted in a geriatric patient, both the patient and her responsible relatives should be thoroughly informed that the pessary was inserted and that regular office visits—no less frequent than every 2 months—will be mandatory. Geriatric patients are likely to forget, and a neglected pessary may not be discovered until years later, when it has ulcerated into the bladder or rectum. At each office visit the pessary should be removed and cleaned. The vaginal mucosa should be inspected for ulceration prior to its insertion. Vaginal douches may be required for the vaginal discharge that regularly occurs. The use of estrogen vaginal creams promotes stimulation of the vaginal mucosa and aids in the prevention of ulceration. Some patients or members of the family may be taught to remove the pessary at bedtime and replace it in the morning. Although this is the best practice, it may not be possible with a geriatric patient.

In summary, the unique ways the urethra and bladder are affected by postmenopausal changes in the aging female, particularly in the "old" geriatric patient, make geriatric gynecology an important aspect of geriatric medicine. Gynecologic examination in women this age should not be neglected.

9

PREVENTION AND OPERATIVE TREATMENT OF RELAXATIONS AND LACERATIONS OF THE POSTERIOR VAGINA AND PERINEUM:
1. CHOICE OF EPISIOTOMY
2. POSTERIOR COLPOPERINEOPLASTY

BROOKS RANNEY, M.D.

Posterior colpoperineoplasty is needed more often than any other vaginoplasty procedure. The gynecologic operator must guard against tight or rigid suturing, which can produce either introital or vaginal narrowing, and may cause subsequent dyspareunia. Such scarring is difficult to correct later.[1-5] However, if sutures are placed carefully, with the constant aim of providing support without constriction, the long-term result will usually be both comfort and physiologic function of both the vagina and the rectum.

In this report, we will discuss 1) the obstetric causes of rectal, anal, and perineal scarring and stretching, and techniques for their prevention; 2) the occurrence of symptomatic rectoceles; 3) methods of posterior colpoperineoplasty which may be adapted to each patient's respective lacerations or relaxations; and 4) the long-term results which we have observed.

Causes and General Occurrence of Rectocele and Perineal Lacerations

Obstetric Causes and Their Partial Prevention

Some stretching and tearing of the endopelvic fascia and the *upper two thirds* of the rectovaginal septum usually occur during any obstetric labor, depending upon the health and elasticity of the supporting tissues, the size of the fetus traversing the birth canal, the duration of labor, the amount of strenuous bearing down which the mother performs, the precipitate speed of the second stage of labor, and the need for obstetric manipulations. Conversely, the perineum and adjacent supporting structures can be well protected from stretching and tearing during the latter part of labor and delivery by properly chosen episiotomies performed as the fetal head begins to distend the perineum, but before the perineal tissues have been severely stretched or torn.

If the fetal head is small or moderate in size, if the mother's perineal body is of average height and thickness, if the supporting tissues are elastic, and if the delivery is performed spontaneously or by the use of outlet forceps, a median episiotomy may be chosen. It probably will provide sufficient space for delivery without jeopardizing the anal sphincter or the rectum. Median episiotomies usually may be sutured more rapidly than mediolateral episiotomies, requiring less skill, using fewer sutures, and permitting less blood loss; they often heal with less temporary perineal discomfort. However, even after careful suturing and good healing, the perineal body is often narrower at its base, following median episiotomy, than it is following mediolateral episiotomy, so that the pelvic floor is not always well protected by this procedure. Moreover, median episiotomies can extend through the anal sphincter or into the rectum much more commonly than mediolateral episiotomies during delivery.[6-11] In spite of the excellent perineal blood supply and careful suturing, not all patients who have had third- or fourth-degree perineal incisions or lacerations will heal well. In many, the perineal body will heal thinly, providing poor support. A large number will have permanent scar in the rectal wall which may tear repeatedly if they become constipated, resulting in uncomfortable anterior anal fissures. A smaller number will experience inadequate healing of the anal sphincter, causing anal incontinence if the stool is soft, and a few will heal so poorly that rectovaginal fistulas form which require subsequent repair.

If the obstetrician chooses inaccurately by performing a median episiotomy just before obstetric delivery, and it becomes apparent that during delivery the median episiotomy is likely to extend into the rectal sphincter or beyond, then the obstetrician may push the fetal head gently upwards, and quickly angulate the apex of the episiotomy diagonally to one side with a scissors, changing it into a "hockey-stick," mediolateral episiotomy. This simple procedure will avoid lacerating the anal sphincter or rectum. If one is well acquainted with the perineal anatomy, anatomic repair of this unusual mediolateral episiotomy is not much more difficult than that of a standard mediolateral episiotomy.

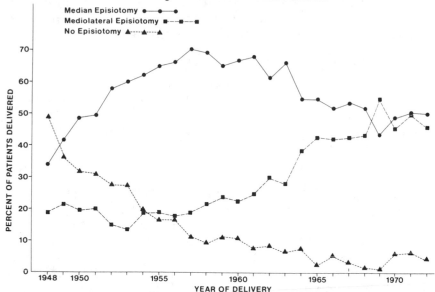

Episiotomy and Repair during Obstetric Delivery
(4721 Vaginal Deliveries of Viable Babies)

Median Episiotomy ●——●——●
Mediolateral Episiotomy ■——■——■
No Episiotomy ▲----▲----▲

PERCENT OF PATIENTS DELIVERED

YEAR OF DELIVERY

However, for the obstetric patient with a large fetus, for operative deliveries, for patients who have short or rigid perineums, for patients whose tissues are inelastic, and for some primigravidas, it is best initially to choose mediolateral episiotomies. Usually, one may avoid damaging the anus or rectum. It takes more time and skill to suture a mediolateral episiotomy. There is a moderate increase in healing time following mediolateral episiotomy, and there is a longer interval of perineal discomfort for the patient. However, the perineal anatomy and support return closer to normal following healing of a mediolateral episiotomy, and function of the rectum and vagina tend to remain more physiological.

Using these concepts during delivery of more than 7,000 obstetric patients, the author has never permitted a fourth-degree perineal laceration to occur. Moreover, none of the patients has experienced subsequent anal incontinence or rectovaginal fistulas. Of 4,721 obstetric patients delivered vaginally of viable babies, however, 19 had some third-degree extensions of episiotomies involving parts of anal sphincters (0.4%). All anal sphincters and perineums were carefully sutured, and healed well; these patients had good subsequent bowel function.

Graph 1 illustrates the method of caring for the perineum during vaginal delivery of 4,721 obstetric patients delivered by the author from 1948 to 1972. During the first decade (1948–1958), we saw a number of patients who had had prior deliveries at home or in nursing homes. Their perineums were stretched, torn, and lacerated, so that episiotomy was a useless and unnecessary procedure. During the last fifteen years of the study, about 95% of obstetric patients had their perineums protected by the use of either median or medio-lateral episiotomies and repairs. From 1963 to the end of the study, a notable increase in the percent of mediolateral episiotomies coincided with a similar increase in the percent of primigravida patients who were delivered by the author.

Other Contributing Causes

During the late menstrual years and after the menopause, estrogen levels in most women decrease. Since estrogens are a growth hormone for most of the pelvic structures, and partic-ularly for elastic tissues in the pelvic region, diminished levels cause pelvic supporting structures to become less elastic, and to sag more, so that previous tearing and relaxations due to childbirth often become more perceptible and symptomatic at this time. Similarly, uterine retrodisplacement allows the uterus to descend more readily through the vaginal sleeve and can aggravate pelvic relaxations. The effect of gravity causes relaxations to become worse. Heavy work, straining during passage of bowel movements, and repeated coital stretching may also aggravate pelvic relaxations.

In rare instances, women may develop posterior vaginal relaxations without prior childbirth stretching. Very likely, these result from either inherited or nutritional deficiencies of the supporting tissues.

General Occurrence

During the thirty-five years 1948–1983, among 3,757 pa-tients who required major gynecologic operations by the author, 1,382 (36.8%) have needed posterior colpoperineoplas-ties to correct symptomatic rectoceles, perineal relaxations, perineal lacerations, or incompetent anal sphincters.

Parity

Among the 1,382 patients who needed posterior colpoperi-neoplasty, only 6 (0.4%) had never been married, and only 14 others (1%) had never had a baby delivered vaginally. All 20 of these patients had partial prolapse of the uterus and other vaginal relaxations, suggesting poor tissue integrity. Each of

TABLE 1. EFFECTS OF PRIOR DELIVERY TECHNIQUES UPON SUBSEQUENT PERINEAL SUPPORT

Extent of Perineal Laceration	Numbers of Old Perineal Lacerations	
	1948-1963 Mostly Home Deliveries 565 Patients	1964-1983 Mostly Hospital Deliveries 817 Patients
1st degree	86	53
2nd degree	186	47
3rd degree	156	12
4th degree	40	2
TOTALS	468 = 82.8%	114 = 13.9%

the remaining 1,362 patients had had between 1 and 16 vaginal deliveries (average - 4.15 deliveries).

Age

At the time of posterior colpoperineoplasty, the youngest patient was only 25 years old. She had had three babies and suffered from procidentia. The oldest patient was 89. She lived and benefited from her operative repair for five more years, dying from a cardiac cause at age 94. Most patients were between 40 and 65; the average age was 53.5 years.

Anatomical Distortions Related to Techniques during Prior Obstetric Deliveries

Most patients upon whom we performed posterior colpoperineoplasties during the years 1948-1963 had had one or many prior home deliveries supervised by other physicians (Table 1). The resultant old perineal relaxations are listed by degrees in Table 1. It is noteworthy that 40 of these old lacerations were fourth-degree, and 156 were third-degree tears.

Conversely, many patients operated upon during the years 1964-1983 had been delivered previously in the obstetric department of a community hospital by the author or his associates. Most perineums had been protected by individually chosen episiotomies and repairs. When circumstances indicated, fetal heads had been gently delivered, using outlet forceps. As a result, only 114 of these 817 gynecologic patients had any notable perineal lacerations or relaxations, of which 53 were merely first-degree lacerations, and 47 were only second-degree lacerations. Thus most of these 817 patients needed only minimal perineoplasties.

Symptoms and Findings

It is possible to protect the perineum with reasonable consistency during obstetric delivery; however, the mid and upper portions of the rectovaginal septum cannot be protected from stretching as a fetus passes through the birth canal. Thereafter, this weakened rectovaginal septum bulges quite freely into the vagina, and even out through the vulva, whenever women must strain to pass firm bowel movements. Indeed, patients with large rectoceles must support the vaginal ballooning, using their hands, to achieve bowel movements. The severe straining to pass stool engorges veins around the rectum, causing painful "hemorrhoids." Large ballooned masses of feces, which are forced through the anus, cause lacerations of the anal mucosa. Recurring fissuring, healing, and scarring can produce anal stenosis. Patients who have had third- and fourth-degree obstetric lacerations of the perineum, and who already have a scar in the rectal or anal mucosa, are more prone to develop "fissuring" in this region.

All 1,382 of the reported patients had symptomatic rectoceles. Painful bowel movements were reported by 805 patients. Recurring rectal bleeding was reported by 254 patients. In 96 patients, there was sufficient anal stenosis to interfere with the passage of a normal-sized stool.

In 65 patients (4.7%), previous posterior colpoperineoplasty, performed elsewhere, had provided a degree of improved bowel function, but had resulted in painful dyspareunia, caused by too much narrowing and scarring of the vagina.[1-5] In some, the painful narrowing was introital and had been caused by suturing together the posterior aspects of the labia minora. However, most of this painful narrowing was near or just above the hymen, and had been caused by dense scar and constriction, which resulted from rigid suturing together of large sweeps of levator ani muscle. This surgical technique causes a "transverse bar," or a "washboard perineum." Such scar almost always interferes with comfortable coitus.[5,12]

Techniques of Posterior Colpoperineoplasty:

Preparation

If there is anal stenosis, the anal sphincter and scar should be dilated slowly and carefully with two lubricated fingers of the gloved hand immediately after induction of anesthesia, and before performing the preoperative vaginal preparation.

Dissection

In patients who have symptomatic rectoceles, but whose perineums remain essentially intact, one may make the initial incision by depressing and stretching laterally the tissues of the fourchette, using two fingers of the left hand, and by incising the mucosa and underlying connective tissues quite superficially in the midline with a scalpel (Fig. 1). Then an Allis forceps is placed on the incised mucosa, each side, midway between the mucocutaneous junction and the hymenal ring.

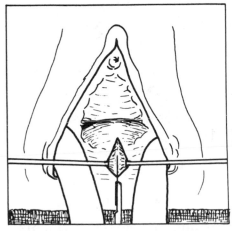 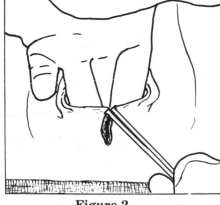

Figure 1.   Figure 2.

Conversely, if there has been a significant degree of old perineal laceration, the gynecologist must immediately estimate how much perineal buildup will be optimal during the later suturing. Based upon this estimate, an Allis forceps is placed on each side, midway between the mucocutaneous junction and the hymenal ring. In some patients who have asymmetrical postobstetric scars, careful individual judgment is needed to adapt the initial placement of Allis forceps. If two or three fingers of the left hand are placed in the vagina, and the tips of the forceps are held together around those fingers (Fig. 2), one can estimate the postoperative introital capacity, and can then readjust the Allis forceps as needed prior to the initial incision.

A flat V is incised with a scalpel, on perineal skin, between the Allis forceps; the depth of the V varies with the patient. A flat diamond of introital mucosa may be discarded (Fig. 3). Then the Allis forceps are reapplied to the lateral borders of the incised mucosa.

If the patient has had a third-degree or fourth-degree laceration of the perineum, then an inverted, U-shaped, Warren flap[13] of posterior vaginal mucosa may be incised with a scalpel, starting lateral to the dimple which connotes one healed edge of the old anal sphincter laceration, and continu-

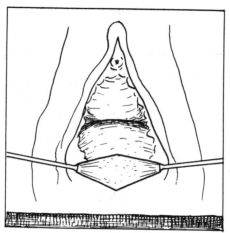

Figure 3.

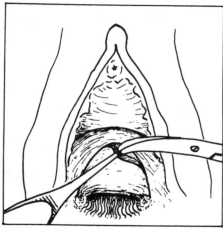

Figure 4.

ing around to a similar point on the opposite side (Fig. 4). This flap of vaginal mucosa is dissected down carefully, without defects, so that subsequent sutures will be protected from fecal contamination from the rectum and anus. Before reconstruction of the perineum, the scarred ends of the old laceration of the anal sphincter should be dissected free laterally, identified, and approximated with several interrupted sutures (Fig. 5). After perineal reconstruction, the skin-mucosal closure on the perineum will be an inverted Y. (Alternatively, in some patients who have old fourth-degree lacerations, the Noble-Mengert repair[2,14] will adapt better to the residual tissues; then the skin-mucosal closure will be an inverted T-shape, but will be somewhat closer to the anus.)

The posterior vaginal mucosa is alternately dissected and incised carefully, one centimeter at a time, using scissors, while successive pairs of Kocher forceps stretch mucosal borders apart, up, and away from the underlying perineal scar and the lower half of the rectocele (Fig. 6). This incision extends no higher than half way up to the vaginal vault. Then an Allis forceps is clamped on the apex (Fig. 7).

Using the Kocher forceps for traction on the mucosa, and using a tissue forceps for countertraction on the underlying scar and connective tissue, the latter may be dissected away from the perineal skin and vulvar and vaginal mucosa with dissecting scissors, by alternately snipping and spreading the blades of the scissors (Fig. 7). The individually variable breadth of dissection is that which is estimated to be necessary for subsequent support of the rectal wall when sutured, but no further, to avoid painful vaginal constriction. This is

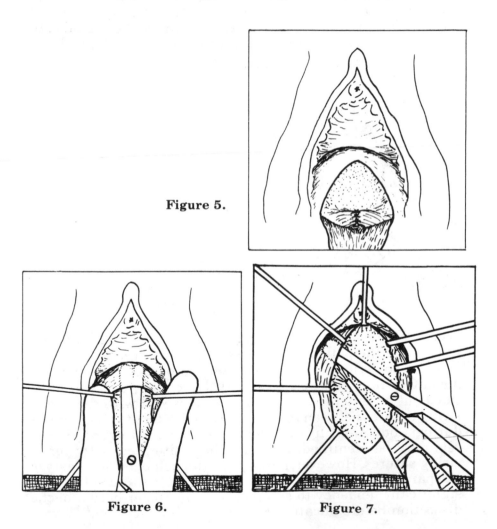

Figure 5.

Figure 6.

Figure 7.

accomplished first on one side, then on the other. Little perineal dissection is needed if there has been little perineal relaxation.

When the dissection has extended above the perineum and above the old obstetric scar, one finds a loose seam of areolar tissue between the rectum and the vagina.[15] At this time the rectal wall can be most proficiently separated from the vaginal wall by rolling a gauze sponge into a ball between the rectum and the upper vagina, using finger pressure downward, while the operative assistants retract straight upward on the Allis forceps and the two Kocher forceps which were previously placed near the apex of the vaginal mucosal incision (Fig. 8). This sponge dissection should be extended to the estimated upper border of the rectocele, which should have

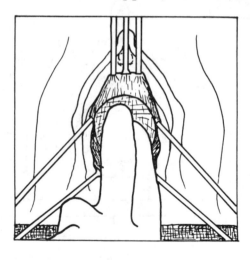

Figure 8.

been evaluated preoperatively, during rectovaginal examination, while the patient was awake and straining down.

If the posterior colpoperineoplasty is being performed immediately following a vaginal hysterectomy, one will have ruled out an enterocele, or will have closed it with the pursestring sutures between the uterosacral ligaments.[16] Similarly, during abdominal hysterectomy, tendencies toward enterocele may be identified, and may be obliterated with pursestring sutures. However, if this posterior colpoperineoplasty is a separate procedure, one must try to identify and suture any significant tendency to enterocele at the upper border of the dissection before plicating the rectovaginal septum.[3-5,16]

The perineal, rectal, and vaginal tissues tend to be highly vascular. Arterial bleeders and larger venous bleeders should be clamped and ligated delicately to avoid rectal trauma. Most larger bleeders may be avoided if the dissection is not carried too far laterally, where it may involve branches of the inferior hemorrhoidal arteries.

Suturing

Posterior colpoperineoplasty consists of two parts: first, one must correct the rectocele; then one must construct an adequate, functional perineum.

Rectocele: To correct the rectocele, one must plicate the "rectovaginal fascia," which is really the muscularis of the rectal wall plus some attenuated fibers of the endopelvic fascia.[15]

Several basic principles should be kept in mind:

a) To promote hemostasis and to limit bulky suture knots; a continuous suture is preferable to interrupted sutures.

b) To eliminate "dead space" in which blood and serum may otherwise accumulate; this suture should also be sewn into the vaginal mucosa, above.

c) Some redundancy of the anterior rectal wall, which may bulge into the rectum, is certain to be produced by the suturing. It is preferable that this redundancy be drawn *high* in the rectum, rather than that it be allowed to sag down near the anus, where it might produce symptoms of a large, anterior hemorrhoid. Therefore, the rectocele plication should be sewn up under the *intact* vaginal mucosa of the upper *vagina.*

d) To avoid rectal trauma and to avoid later rigid scar, frequent, small, superficial stitches are preferable to a few, large, strangulating "sweeps" of tissue.

e) Because of the potential danger of fecal contamination of a stitch, which might inadvertently penetrate too close to the rectal lumen, we prefer to use 0 catgut which will slough early at a contaminated point, rather than use the synthetic, absorbable sutures here, which might persist longer to create a fistula.

By using one or two fingers to depress and stretch the bulging rectocele (Fig. 9), one may visualize and suture its upper border directly to the adjacent, upper vaginal mucosa. A knot anchors this suture. Then, using many small superficial stitches taken in a deep U-shape over the rectocele, successive circles of the redundant "rectovaginal fascia" are gathered cephalad and tacked up to the intact vaginal mucosa. This is repeated until all or most of the rectocele has been gathered up

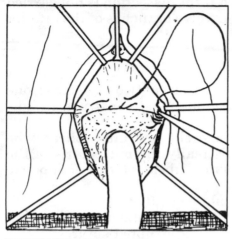

Figure 9.

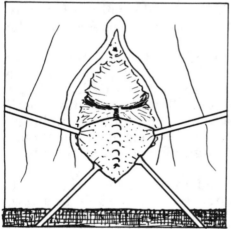

Figure 10.

by plication, and has been sutured up *under intact vaginal mucosa.* Continuing with the same suture, but now using tissue forceps to maneuver structures, the lower rectovaginal fascia is plicated. The suture is finally sewn into significant perineal connective tissues, and then is tied (Fig. 10). This running suture builds a flexibly firm, rectal ceiling, which replaces the "balloon" of the old rectocele. Thereafter, the fecal stream is directed toward the anus.

The vaginal mucosa is seldom trimmed and then only slightly, because it may be needed to cover the reconstructed introitus. It is sutured to underlying connective tissue, using #0 Dexon in a continuous, vertical, tension-approximation suture, which neatly everts and approximates the mucosal borders, and eliminates most of the underlying "dead space."

This mucosal suture is interrupted once, twice, or more times; the assistant holds firm tension on it, while one, two, or more successive rows of interrupted V-type 0 catgut sutures are placed to build the perineum up to the breadth and height needed to provide good support without later dyspareunia (Fig. 11). Sutures which cause much perineal height, without enough depth at the base, will produce a "dashboard perineum,"[2] which is like a Hollywood facade; it may look good on

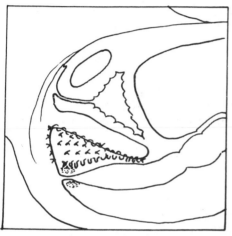
Figure 11.

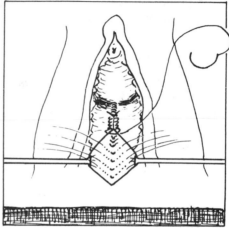
Figure 12.

the outside, but will have little depth or functional capacity! In general, the depth and height of perineal suturing depends upon the prior degree of integrity of the perineum, that is, more relaxation—more suturing. Here, again, meticulous suturing is individually adapted to the scarred tissues of each perineum. One should not reach out widely with sutures to obtain large bits of the levator ani muscle, because the resulting rigid tightness will often cause later perineal pain or dyspareunia.[1-5] During all suturing, frequent palpation of the contour, diameter, depth, and flexibility of the vagina with two or three fingers gives the operator information which cannot be obtained by any other method (Fig. 12).

Interrupted fine silk sutures are used to close the perineal skin, because subcuticular, absorbable sutures in the perineal skin do not heal as well in the gynecologic patient as they do in the postpartum patient. These fine silk sutures are not removed until the patient's first postoperative visit to the office, in order to protect against inadvertent separation and broad scarring of the perineal skin, which may result when the skin has been closed with rapidly absorbable sutures, or when the skin sutures are removed before the patient leaves the hospital.

The 66 patients who had had painful vaginal or introital narrowing from prior posterior colpoperineoplasties were treated by individually adapted modifications of perineotomy—that is, vertical incision and transverse suturing. In all of these 66 patients, other areas of the rectovaginal septum and/or perineum remained relaxed, and also needed supportive repair.

After posterior colpoperineoplasty, a vaginal pack is inserted to press the vaginal mucosa gently against underlying connective tissues; this is removed in 24 hours. A Foley catheter drains the bladder for two or three days; this catheter is needed longer if an anterior colpoplasty was also performed.

Associated Operative Procedures, Follow-up, and Long-Term Results

Associated Operative Procedures

Among these 1,382 patients who needed posterior colpoperineoplasties, 711 were performed in association with vaginal hysterectomy, and 442 in association with abdominal hysterectomy. Prior subtotal hysterectomy had been performed for 42 of these patients; therefore, the residual cervical stumps were removed just prior to this posterior colpoperineoplasty. Prior total hysterectomies had been performed for 112 of these patients, who then needed vaginoplasties from one to twenty years later. At the time of their posterior colpoperineoplasties, 511 of these patients needed repairs of their enteroceles, 728 needed anterior colpoplasties, and 46 needed anterior bladder-neck suspensions.

Follow-up

Among these 1,382 patients upon whom we have performed posterior colpoperineoplasties, 943 (68.2%) have been followed by periodic examinations until the end of this study, for intervals ranging from 35 years down to one year (average, 14.2 years). Another 133 patients (9.6%) received full follow-up by periodic examinations until their deaths, which occurred from 33 years down to two years after their respective operations. Ages at death ranged from 30 to 94, the average age of death being 74.1 years. Causes of death were cardiac disease, 48; stroke, 41; cancer, 30; other causes, 16. The remaining 306 patients (22.1%) had partial follow-up by periodic examinations from one to 25 years after their posterior colpoperineoplasties.

Long-Term Results

Based upon subsequent history and pelvic and rectal examinations, most of these patients had satisfactory function of the lower bowel and vagina after their operations. Only 14 patients (1%) needed any subsequent operation of the posterior vaginal wall or perineum, sometime between 10 and 21 years after their posterior colpoperineoplasties. Symptomatic high rectoceles, above the previous vaginoplasties, developed in nine patients. These might have been avoided by extending the initial vaginoplasty higher. Enteroceles developed in three. Possibly, these could have been recognized and repaired initially.[16] One patient needed a perineotomy to enlarge a painful introitus. Only one patient needed a subsequent hemorrhoidectomy.

Complications and their Prevention

There were only two significant early complications which resulted from posterior colpoperineoplasty in these 1,382 patients—one uncommon, and the other rare. Since the vagina is so close to the anus, it is usually contaminated by microorganisms from the bowel, especially if the perineum has been shortened by an old laceration. Preoperatively, we attempt to decrease vaginal contamination with douches and sulfa cream in the vagina the night before the operation, and with pHisoHex preparation just before operation. Also, we use appropriate antibiotics, starting preoperatively and continuing for variable intervals postoperatively, depending upon the postoperative course of the patient. In addition, postmenopausal women receive estrogens postoperatively to improve blood supply and nutrition to the healing tissues. As a result of these precautions, postoperative infections have been uncommon, healing has almost always been primary, and our patients have had no postoperative rectovaginal fistulas.

The rare complication is that of delayed arterial hemorrhage from the vagina, caused by separation of the healing mucosal borders of the posterior colpoperineoplasty, usually occurring between ten days and three weeks after operation as the catgut sutures soften. The patient usually notices this bleeding immediately after passage of a very firm bowel movement which may distend the healing posterior wall and cause separation of the mucosa. Identification of the separated, bleeding mucosa and placement of interrupted figure-of-8 sutures constitutes the necessary emergency treatment. Since our fifth such delayed hemorrhage (0.36%), we have chosen #0 Dexon for the initial closure of the posterior vaginal mucosa, tacking the mucosa to underlying connective tissue. Since Dexon absorbs more slowly than catgut sutures and holds perhaps a week longer, it permits greater healing before separation of the absorbable suture material. Since Dexon #0 has been used, there have been no more delayed hemorrhages.

Coitus should be avoided for at least two months postoperatively. Earlier coital stretching may disrupt suture lines and can cause severe postcoital hemorrhage.[17]

Comment

During recent years, we have seen increasing instances in which young women have either lacerated anal sphincters or rectums, or these structures have been cut through during obstetric delivery. Rectal and vaginal mucosa has usually healed, although there have been some rectovaginal fistulas among these patients. However, the anal sphincter apparently does not heal well in some of these patients, because there has been an increasing incidence of anal incontinence of feces. Likewise, there have been perineums which are very thin and non-supportive. Not only does this combination produce uncomfortable and unphysiologic function of the rectum, but it tends to become progressively worse with the passage of time. These observations have convinced us that it is very important, if possible, to preserve the rectum, anus, and rectal sphincter intact during obstetric delivery. At times, the only way to do this is to utilize mediolateral episiotomy.

It is apparent to physicians who have learned from years of both obstetric and gynecologic experience that the presently recurring overemphasis of propaganda (which implies that a mother is at least a partial failure if she doesn't push her baby out of the birth canal, regardless of cephalopelvic dimensions, uterine inertia, or other soft-tissue dystocia) will cause more

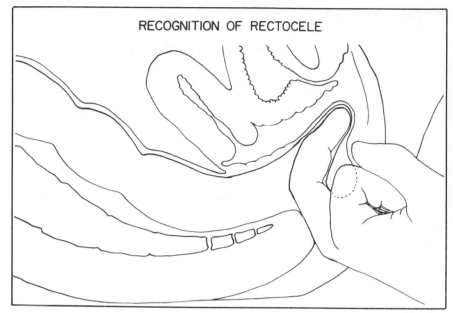

RECOGNITION OF RECTOCELE

Figure 13.

women to develop painful and uncomfortable pelvic relaxations, so that more women will be needing vaginoplasties as they grow older. These problems can be avoided by careful, knowledgeable, and considerate obstetric deliveries.

If a parous woman complains of difficult or painful bowel movements, "rectal bleeding," or hemorrhoids," she should be checked for rectocele (Fig. 13). If she has a rectocele, it will cause her to strain to pass her bowel, and this will produce all of the symptoms noted above. After ruling out tumors or other pathology of the bowel, such a patient should not have a hemorrhoidectomy or another anal procedure, which would be similar to treating a symptom. Rather, she should have a posterior colpoperineoplasty to eliminate her bulging rectocele, which will treat the basic cause of her troubles, and help her to have physiologic bowel movements. Then, the anal symptoms usually will resolve spontaneously. If not, the anus can be operated upon later. It is not wise to operate on both sides of the perineal body at the same time, because of the danger of fistula formation.

Among the various vaginoplasties, patients derive their most consistent symptomatic and functional benefits from indicated and individually adapted posterior colpoperineoplasty. Most patients will be gratified by the markedly improved function of the rectum and anus which they will note during the first postoperative bowel movement. If the operator is experienced and skillful, if his judgment has been good, and if he has carefully avoided overcorrection of the perineum,[1,3-5,12,18] then, after healing is complete or about eight weeks postoperatively, many patients will note satisfactory sexual function of the vagina and the introitus. There are few operative procedures which can provide so much comfort and improved function with so slight a risk.

REFERENCES

1. Jeffcoate TNA. Posterior colpoperineoplasty. Am J Obstet Gynecol 77: 490, 1959.
2. Mengert WF. Complete perineal tear and perineorrhaphy. Clin Obstet Gynecol 4:168, 1961.
3. Symmonds RE, Sheldon RS. Vaginal prolapse after hysterectomy. Obstet Gynecol 25:61, 1965.
4. Pratt JH. Secondary operations to correct failures of previous operations for genital prolapse. Clin Obstet Gynecol 9:1084, 1966.
5. Pratt JH. Surgical repair of rectocele and perineal lacerations. Clin Obstet Gynecol 15:1160, 1972.
6. Cunningham CG, Pilkington JW. Complete perineotomy. Am J Obstet Gynecol 70:1225, 1955.
7. Schelin EC. Discussion of "Complete Perineotomy." Am J Obstet Gynecol 70:1229, 1955.
8. Park J. Discussion of "Complete Perineotomy." Am J Obstet Gynecol 70:1230, 1955.
9. Fleming A. Complete perineotomy. Obstet Gynecol 16:172, 1960.
10. Brantley JT, Burwell, JG. A study of fourth-degree perineal lacerations and their sequelae. Am J Obstet Gynecol 80:711, 1960.
11. Rabins S. Discussion of "A Study of Fourth-degree Perineal Lacerations." Am J Obstet Gynecol 80:713, 1960.
12. Ranney B. Sequelae of incomplete gynecologic operations: IV. The vagina. SD J Med 31:11, 1978.
13. Warren JC. A new method of operation for the relief of rupture of the perineum through the sphincter and rectum. J Am Gynecol Soc 72:322, 1882.
14. Mengert WF. Fish SA. Anterior rectal wall advancement. Obstet Gynecol 5:262, 1955.
15. Curtis AH, Anson BJ, Beaton LE. The anatomy of the subperitoneal tissues and ligamentous structures in relation to surgery of the female pelvic viscera. Surg Gynecol Obstet 70:643, 1940.
16. Ranney B. Enterocele, vaginal prolapse, pelvic hernia. Am J Obstet Gynecol 140:53, 1981.
17. Ranney B. Postoperative vaginal-vault disruption. Obstet Gynecol 23: 793, 1964.
18. DeCosta EJ. Dance me loose. Obstet Gynecol 6:120, 1955.

10

MANAGEMENT OF PELVIC SUPPORT LOSS IN THE GERIATRIC FEMALE

WAYNE F. BADEN, M.D., TOM WALKER, M.D.

Ours is an aging population, with geriatric females far exceeding males. Data from the United States Bureau of Census (1981)[17] reveal that in 1950 there were 6,541,000 women 65 or more years of age. By 1960 their numbers had risen to 9,056,000 and by 1970 to 11,605,000. In 1980 the figures were 15,242,000 geriatric women to 10,303,000 men. On the average, either sex has a life expectancy of 15 years at age 65, 10 years at age 75 and 7½ years at age 85.[14] Increasingly, women are reluctant to tolerate prolapse, urinary incontinence and other major problems of pelvic support loss "just because they are women." Rather, more are opting for an improved quality of life through vaginal reparative procedures. Tancer[16] reviewed 130 patients with elective repair procedures, concluding 15 years ago that when the special needs of these older patients were met, elective gynecologic surgery might be undertaken without regard to the patient's age. There was no mortality and the morbidity was acceptable. Harbrecht et al.[6] reaffirmed that management in the elderly required the usual principles of good surgery along with a special effort to avoid the first mistake in judgment or technical error, especially in patients over 80 years of age.

A number of questions arise. Is age alone, or are the common complications of aging, a contraindication to surgery? Do geriatric women tolerate surgery as well, have more postoperative complications, have more severe defects, have more difficult repairs or have more recurrences than their younger sisters? Might reparative surgery prevent, or at least delay, their need for nursing home care? In short, should they and their gynecologists be encouraged or discouraged from undertaking reparative procedures?

In search of answers to these and other questions, the authors reviewed their reparative procedures in women 65 or more years (Group 65+), performed between January 1, 1970 and July 1, 1982. Forty-four such patients with ages ranging from 65 to 83, averaging 70.5 years, were found with adequate data. These patients were matched for defect types and reparative procedures with 44 patients ranging from 24 to 39 years of age, averaging 33.7 years. All patients had had routine history and physical examination; most had had preoperative evaluation with their internist. The anesthesiology consultation was essentially routine, and additional consultants were used liberally. Pelvic examination included grading each of the six vaginal sites along the vaginal canal from 0-4, evaluation of the posterior urethrovesical angle (PUVA) and subpubic urethral rotation, and determination of urethral, vesical or rectal detachments from their normal supportive structures. Symptoms were correlated with the sites involved. During the late 1970s, urethrocystoscopy and urodynamic studies on urinary incontinent patients were nearly routine. These tests were later performed primarily upon indication, as confidence in physical diagnosis and history grew. Little effect was recorded on the cure rates. Almost all patients with major reparative procedures received antibiotics, usually during their entire hospital stay. Followup examinations were correlated with the preoperative evaluation, and each site was again graded from 0-4. Posterior urethrovesical angle, subpubic urethral rotation, various detachments and relief of symptoms were correlated with preoperative status. Patients were followed at six weeks, six months and then annually for as long as 13 years maximum.

Fundamentals

Pelvic support loss may be defined as inadequate or abnormal supportive tissues at one or more sites along the vaginal canal. These sites are the urethral (urethrocele) and bladder (cystocele) in the anterior, the uterine (prolapse) and culdesac (enterocele) in the superior, and the rectal (rectocele) and perineal (chronic perineal laceration) sites in the posterior vaginal segments. The common symptoms are urinary incontinence, urinary retention, falling out, pelvic pressure, bowel pocketing and anal incontinence. Most gynecologists are well aware that the more severe the support loss, the more difficult the repair and the more likely a postoperative recurrence. These supportive defects usually involve multiple sites, segments and defect types. Because cystocele may occur without urethrocele, prolapse without chronic perineal laceration and so on, the capability for evaluating each individual site independently is essential. Because the defects are usually caused by stress (parturition and menopausal residuae in particular) and are usually in proportion to that stress, they

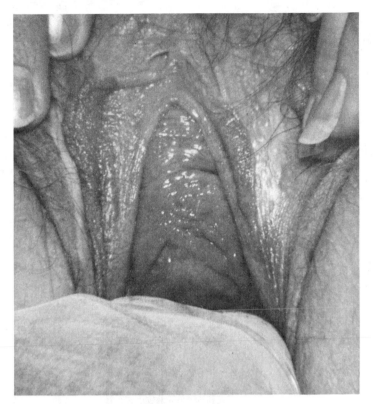

Figure 10:1a. Grading Defect Severity and Defect Diagnosis (Straining).

Grading Defect Severity: One or two fingers are inserted into the vaginal canal, the perineum is gently depressed for better vision, the patient is asked to take a deep breath and strain down firmly and the fingers are slowly withdrawn, as the examiner observes "what falls out and how far." This patient might be graded very simply or very completely, as:

Worst Site: Urethrocele, grade 3 (descent past the hymen).

Worst Segment: Anterior Vaginal Segment (AVS) Profile of 3 2.

Urethrocele, grade 3 and Cystocele, grade 2 (descent to hymen).

The entire Vaginal Profile is 3 2—1 0—1 1 (not all visible).

Urethral Bladder—Uterine Culdesac—Rectocele Perineal Sites.

Defect Diagnosis: Straining descent with subpubic urethral rotation and reversal of the Posterior Urethrovesical Angle (PUVA) indicates damage to the Pubourethral Ligament Complex (PULC: posterior, middle and anterior) and to the paraurethral endopelvic fascia along the Anterior Levator Lines (ALL), where Pubococcygeal Muscles originate from the posterior pubic bones. The bladder descent indicates additional paravesical damage along the Lateral Levator Lines (LLL or Tendinous arches), where lateral vaginal walls attach to lateral pelvic walls. The presence of normal vaginal wall rugae rules out midline and pre- or postcervical fascial sheath damage. Straining medial movement of the Lateral Vaginal Grooves (LVG) and vaginal walls (not seen) was additional evidence of the lateral defects. Superior and posterior vaginal supports were not remarkable.

must be evaluated for their severity under stress.

Since we were unable to find such a method in the literature and in response to these requirements, we developed the Half-way Grading System (HWGS) (Fig. 1a) for evaluating the support loss from 0-4 at all six of the vaginal sites.[1-5] The examiner inserts one or two fingers well into the vagina, gently depresses the perineum to better observe, has the patient take a deep breath and strain down firmly, slowly withdraws the fingers and watches "what falls out and how far." Prolapse (uterine or vaginal cuff) is ideally suited to the method, but straining descent of the posterior urethral, bladder and rectal sites also adapt nicely, as follows:

Grading Descent of Posterior Urethra, Bladder, Uterus and Rectum (straining)
> Grade 0: Normal. No significant descent.
> Grade 1: Descent half-way to the hymeneal line.
> Grade 2: Descent on to the hymeneal line.
> Grade 3: Descent on half-way past the hymen.
> Grade 4: Maximum descent possible at each respective site.

Grading Perineal Laceration is as follows:
> Grade 0: Normal. Little more than hymeneal laceration.
> Grade 1: Laceration half-way to the anal sphincter.
> Grade 2: Laceration to, but not through, the sphincter.
> Grade 3: Laceration through the sphincter.
> Grade 4: Laceration involving rectal mucosa.

Enterocele is difficult to diagnose, let alone grade, but if it is defined as dissection *between* rectal and vaginal walls, grading becomes possible. Note that enterocele is NOT simply prolapse of a relatively normal culdesac. Note, also, that enterocele and prolapse may or may not occur together. With the cervix resting at the 0 station between the ischial spines, the normal culdesac depth is about two centimeters below the uterosacral ligament insertions on the posterior cervix. Essentially, each single grade equals two more centimeters of depth by dissection, as follows:

Grading Enterocele (straining)
> Grade 0: Normal. Two or less centimeters of culdesac depth.
> Grade 1: Rectovaginal dissection 1/4 of the way to the hymen.
> Grade 2: Rectovaginal dissection half-way to the hymen.

Grade 3: Rectovaginal dissection 3/4 of the way to the hymen.

Grade 4: Rectovaginal dissection 4/4 of the way to the hymen.

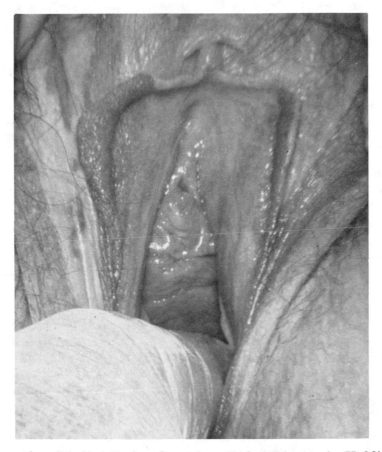

Figure 1b. Grading Defect Severity—Defect Diagnosis (Holding).
The same patient seen in Figure 1a was asked to "hold" (Kegel's pubococcygeal muscle contraction). Although these muscles were firmly contracted, laterally, the urethra and bladder ascend only about halfway to their normal grade 0 level at the line of the vaginal axis. This indicates partial urethrovesical detachment from the pubococcygei muscles. Holding ascent is in proportion to remaining lateral attachment. Total urethro-vesical detachment would have failed to ascend appreciably. Although midline and superior (pre- and postcervical) defects will alter holding ascent, presence of vaginal rugae rules out these defects. Not visible was inadequate upward and lateral retraction of the lateral vaginal walls and LVG with holding, evidence again of the lateral detachments. This patient with only partial urethrovesical detachment might obtain some relief of her urinary incontinence through Kegel's exercises.

The Half-way Grading System, in its simplest form, is used to grade the single worst site along the vaginal tract. When the patient's problems warrant, however, more complete use involves grading the single worst segment or the entire vaginal canal. Used in this manner, the sites are always graded in order: urethral, bladder-uterine, culdesac-rectal and perineal. Grading all six sites in this sequence gives a six-digit Vaginal Profile, which describes the support around the entire vaginal canal and is most useful for research. When a fistula is present, it may be so designated by placing a circle around the grade digit of the involved site.

Concurrently with the HWGS four-point method, a similar clinical evaluation for urinary incontinence was proposed, as follows:

Grading Urinary Incontinence
Grade 0: Normal. No loss of urine.
Grade 1: Loss of a few drops, acceptable to patient and public.
Grade 2: Loss requiring a change of underclothing.
Grade 3: Loss requiring part-time protection.
Grade 4: Loss requiring full-time protection.

We were privileged to work with Kegel[7] for several years. He felt that comparing our straining urethral descent (Fig. 1a) to his holding (pubococcygeal contraction) (Fig. 1b) ascent would further assess the support loss. We should define here the line of the vaginal axis, which is an imaginary line from midhymen to vaginal apex or vault. It was quickly found that straining urethral descent might be followed by negligible, partial or complete failure of holding ascent to the line of the vaginal axis. This failure of ascent has been termed urethral detachment, partial or total, from the lateral, firmly contracted, pubococcygeal muscles. Could we have been plicating healthy midline fascia all these years, not recognizing the true lateral defects? Would this account, at least in part, for the reparative failure rates still as high as 45%[15]? Our first transvaginal, paravaginal, bilateral urethral, reattachment in 1970[3] confirmed these suspicions. Similar detachments of bladder and rectum were later noted and the transvaginal lateral reattachments extended to include these structures. Encouraged by the transvaginal, bilateral, paraurethrovesical and pararectal reattachments, we developed the bilateral paraurethral repair by the abdominal route in 1973. Each progressive technique reaffirmed the validity of lateral, paravaginal defects. We were unaware that paraurethrovesical

PELVIC SUPPORTS
(From Above)

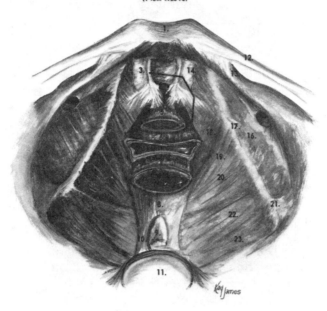

1. Symphysis Pubis	6. Vagina	12. Inguinal Ligament	18. Pubococcygeal M.
2. Internal Pubourethral L.	7. Rectum	13. Cooper's Ligament	19. Endopelvic Fascia
3. Internal Fascia	8. Levator Plate	14. Genital Hiatus Fascia	20. Iliococcygeal M.
Urogenital Diaphragm	9. Coccyx	15. Obturator Foramen	21. Ischial Spine
4. Urethra	10. Anterior Sacrococcygeal L.	16. Obturator Internus M.	22. Coccygeal M.
5. Bladder	11. Sacrum	17. Tendinous Arch	23. Piriformis M.

Figure 10:2. Pelvic Supports from Above.

Key anatomic structures and tissues are shown. The abdominal transversalis fascia crosses the iliopectineal lines, separating false from true pelvic cavities, to become the endopelvic fascia, which covers pelvic muscles and viscera. The Tendinous arches, or Lateral Levator Lines (LLL) mark the origin of the pelvic levator sling from the obturator internus muscles, also denoting the lateral attachment line of the vaginal walls. Anteriorly, the LLL swing medially along the origin of the pubococcygeal portion of the levator muscles from posterior pubic bones, as the Anterior Levator Lines (ALL). The ALL terminates medially at the lateral border of the urogenital hiatus, where pubococcygeal muscle fascia fuses with superior (internal) fascia of the urogenital diaphragm to form the Posterior Pubourethral Ligaments (PPUL), just medial to the number 14. The Superior fascia of the urogenital diaphragm lies between the PPUL, to the right of the number 3. Middle and anterior pubourethral ligaments are not seen. While the black lines indicate the commonest site of paraurethrovesical defects, these defects usually are bilateral and often extend posteriorly to also involve pararectal levels. Defects of the sacrococcygeal insertions of the levator muscles have been described by Nichols,[12] and we have confirmed them by physical diagnosis. Midline defects (not seen) usually involve bladder, central culdesac, rectal and perineal sites. Transverse (pre- and postcervical defects) are also vaginal endopelvic fascial sheath defects (also not visible). Muscle damage often involves pubococcygeal diastasis, but retropubic pubococcygeal muscle lacerations or avulsions do occur.

detachments had been previously reported, and repaired both abdominally and vaginally, by White (1912).[18]

Functional Supportive Anatomy (Figure 2)

Most gynecologists are familiar with normal pelvic anatomy, but much less so with functional supportive defects. A few anatomic features, unique to anatomic restoration, warrant clarification. The obturator internus, coccygeal and piriformis muscles form the lateral pelvic walls. The levator muscles, composed of the pubo- and ilio-coccygeal portions, form the pelvic sling, which is the basic support of the pelvic structures. The levator muscles originate from the postero-lateral pubic bones along the Anterior Levator Lines (ALL), and from the obturator muscles along the Lateral Levator Lines (LLL) (tendinous arches), which extend from postero-lateral pubic bone back to the ischial spine on each side. The levator muscles then swing downward and backward, joining each other in the midline, and finally attaching posteriorly as the Anterior Sacrococcygeal Ligaments. The pelvic sling is perforated by the rectal hiatus posteriorly, and the urogenital hiatus anteriorly. The urethra and vagina pass through the latter hiatus en route to the vulva. Lying between the pubic rami, just external to the pubococcygeal muscles, is the deep transverse perineal muscle, which offers reinforcement to the urogenital hiatus. Bulbocavernosus, superficial transverse perineal and anal sphincter muscles complete the perineal body.

The endopelvic fascia (EPF), which covers the intrapelvic muscles and the pelvic structure, may be conveniently divided into precervical, lateral cervical and postcervical portions. The precervical portion (pubocervical) is attached to the ALL and LLL on either side. The lateral cervical fascia is the lateral cervical ligament (LCL). The postcervical fascia is composed of the central culdesac proper fascia, and the more lateral uterosacral ligament portions, all of which attach cervix to sacral 2, 3 and 4 vertebrae. The cervix normally rests just between the ischial spines (Grade 0 station). Two features are of special importance. First, the vaginal epithelium is surrounded by an endopelvic fascial sheath, which then is attached to anterolateral and posterior sheath supports. The second feature is that the superior fascia of the deep transverse perineal muscle joins with the pubococcygeal muscle fascia, as the latter swings around the medial edge of the muscles (lateral edge of the urogenital hiatus), to form the posterior pubourethral ligament (PPUL).[11] Middle pubourethral ligaments (MPUL) and anterior pubourethral ligaments (APUL) make up the remainder of the pubourethral ligament complex (PULC).

Defects may involve muscles, EPF or both. The commonest muscular defect is midline pubococcygeal diastasis, although lacerations just behind the pubic bones are not uncommon. Nichols[12] has described a loss of attachment of the posterior pelvic sling to the coccyx, and we have confirmed this entity by physical diagnosis. Midline EPF defects have been known for many years. Their midline plication technique has been the standard for anterior and posterior vaginal repair. These defects lie in the vaginal EPF sheath and are termed intrinsic defects. Superior fascial defects involve pre- and post-cervical avulsions, partial or total, from the cervix. These, too, are intrinsic sheath defects. Lateral (extrinsic) defects lie just medial to the ALL and LLL, or involve the Lateral Cervical Ligaments or Uterosacral Ligaments. These detachments of the sheath supports or extrinsic defects are now receiving proper attention. It is obvious that each defect, midline, lateral and superior, will require its own special technique for anatomic restoration. Combinations of these defect types are almost the rule.

Defect Diagnosis (Figures 1a, b)

The recognition and differentiation of midline, lateral and superior defects is readily accomplished. It cannot be over-stressed that the gynecologist must first know the normal before the abnormal will be recognized. The straining descent of the HWGS serves to identify the general severity of the support loss at each of the six vaginal sites. Reversal of the posterior urethrovesical angle (PUVA) and subpubic urethral rotation identify damage to the pubourethral ligament complex (PULC), most often noted with urinary incontinence. When cystocele exceeds urethrocele, the acute PUVA formed is often associated with sluggish bladder function or even total obstruction. The PUVA may be normal, reversed or acute. Normally, *straining* causes little or no cervical descent. The urethra, bladder and rectum merely approximate the line of the vaginal axis. The lateral vaginal grooves (LVG), formed by approximation of anterior and posterior vaginal walls, show no blunting or medial movement. Upon *holding*, the cervix and culdesac again remain essentially stationary, while the lateral vaginal grooves pull upward and laterally, the bladder and urethra ascend slightly, and the PUVA deepens. With defective supports, *straining* descent may involve uterine prolapse, culdesac deepening with postcervical bulging, and descent past the line of the vaginal axis or hymen by posterior urethra, rectum or bladder. Blunting and medial movement of the LVG are noted on *straining* and poor lateral retraction is seen on *holding*. Loss of rugation and smooth vaginal walls accompany intrinsic defects in the vaginal sheath with associated loss of reparative fascia in the involved area. Precervical or postcervical bulging of smooth vaginal walls usually identify pre- or postcervical fascial avulsions, which may blend with anterior cystocele or posterior rectocele. Anterior vaginal segment defects usually involve bilateral detachments, frequent midline fascial damage and often precervical avulsion. Each defect requires its own specific repair. Posterior vaginal segment defects are mostly midline with frequent postcervical and pararectal detachments. Superior defects involve lateral cervical damage and unilateral or bilateral uterosacral ligament avulsions, usually associated with a central enterocele. Perineal defects usually lie midline, although sulcal damage is not uncommon.

Management of Pelvic Support Loss

Non-surgical Management

1. The avoidance of increased intra-abdominal pressure may slow progression of pelvic support loss. Weight reduction for the obese, dietary bulk and stool softeners for the constipated, pulmonary hygiene for the respiratory cripple and other similar measures are all of value. Although the use of estrogens may be equivocal, we often use them in daily doses equivalent to 0.625-1.25 mg. of conjugated estrogens.

2. Kegel's exercises[7] (pubococcygeal "holding") may be helpful in the grade 1 or 2 urinary incontinent patient with partial urethral detachment. Yet often the patient's lack of incentive causes failure to exercise. The grade 3 and 4 urinary incontinent patients have adequate incentive, but the associated total urethral detachment precludes cure. However, their muscles will function better after surgical urethral reattachment, if they have been exercised.

3. "Stressless stress" is a term used to describe the patient who has been conditioned to cough, laugh, sneeze, or otherwise stress, with minimal pressure on the bladder. Upon

noting the stimulation, she contracts both abdominal and pubococcygeal muscles and stresses from the diaphragm up. Never a "belly" laugh. Many patients with grade 1 or 2 urinary incontinence obtain adequate relief in this manner.

4. Pessaries do have a role in management of the geriatric patient, although much less so than in prior years. Their use requires an adequate perineal body to support the pessary that then supports the vaginal canal. Many patients will not accept them, many cannot tolerate their erosive action, and many patients simply cannot be fitted. When used, we prefer a folding pessary the patient can be taught to remove each evening and to replace each morning, prior to arising. When solid pessaries must be used, the Gellhorn seems best suited. Many patients use the pessary only long enough to decide a reparative procedure is preferable.

5. Urethral dilation may be helpful in detecting urethral strictures. Traditional midline fascial plication under such a urethral stricture severely compounds the problem and is to be avoided. Urethral dilation to a French 24-28, in conjunction with surgical paraurethral reattachment, may avoid prolonged catheter need with all of its implications.

6. Urethrocystoscopy and urodynamic studies have a definite role, although probably less so than current literature suggests. We performed these tests almost routinely from 1975 to 1979 on the urinary incontinent patient. Ultimately, we realized that adequate screening of these patients was possible through a few simple questions and observations, and with little or no lessening of the cure rates. However, patients with urge or silent incontinence, inability to stop the urinary stream while voiding, history of bedwetting in the patient or her family, history or findings of neurologic disease, major discrepancy between minimal pelvic support with major grade 3 or 4 urinary incontinence, or prior repair, are all candidates for urethrocystoscopy and urodynamic studies.

Preoperative Management

The gynecologist, internist and anesthesiologist form the basic team, so essential for the often complicated care required by elderly patients. Liberal consultations with other specialists may also be indicated. While the gynecologist can adequately screen essentially healthy young women, medical evaluation and management by the internist offers peace of mind for all concerned in the geriatric group. Armed with the necessary preliminary consultations, the anesthesiologist may then make proper decisions in that area. In general, our anesthesiologists prefer that most necessary medicines be continued up to the time of surgery. A complete blood count, routine urinalysis, electrocardiogram if over age 40, chest x-ray if over age 25, coagulation studies when suspect, electrolyte studies if on diuretics or steroids, diabetic regulation with fasting blood sugar just prior to surgery and endocrine studies, may all be in order. Phospholine iodine or beta-blocking drugs should be continued, but with a highly visible notation to that effect on the patient's chart. Monoamine oxide therapy should be discontinued for two weeks prior to anesthesia, except in emergency. Admission to the hospital should provide adequate time for completion of the necessary studies.

Operative Management

General. Gynecologists are taught to consider the entire patient in evaluating gynecologic problems. Similarly, pelvic problems warrant evaluation of all pelvic structures, not just the genitalia. In the same vein, we feel optimal therapy of pelvic support loss warrants evaluation of the entire vaginal tract supports. Many borderline defects, left uncorrected, have come back to haunt us. When in doubt, it is usually best to repair such defects, along with the major ones. With adequate knowledge of reparative anatomy, the gynecologist usually finds adequate in situ tissues for reparative needs. We have used no foreign body material other than non-absorbable sutures, since 1962, nor have we transplanted tissues from adjacent or other sites. Uterosacral ligaments often retract toward their sacral origins when avulsed from the cervix, but are usually easily identified for anatomic reattachment to cervix or cuff. We would suggest the gynecologist become equally adept at both transvaginal and abdominal routes for most defects, other than those of the posterior vaginal segment. Recognition of the normal supportive tissues is absolutely essential before the abnormal can be identified for correction. Our results have steadily improved since we adopted the "defect detection, defect correction" concept, rather than relying upon traditional midline fascial plication for anterior and posterior vaginal repair. The "tent" theory for vaginal repair is also essential to optimal cure. If the top of the tent caves in, the walls may soon come tumbling after. It is amazing how much anterior and posterior vaginal slack disappears when the vaginal cuff is routinely re-supported at

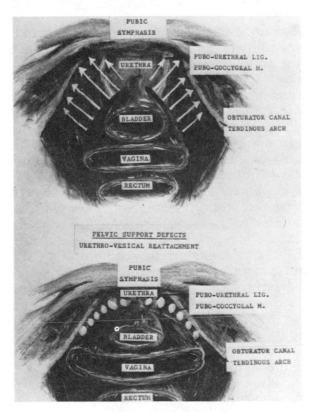

Figure 10:3. Abdominal Bilateral Paraurethrovesical Reattachment.

Above, the patient is in slight reverse Trendelenburg position, the retropubic space has been entered, anteriorly, with blunt finger dissection that has been extended around the pelvic wall to each ischial spine. Urogenital hiatal fat and vessels and obturator canal structures are identified but left relatively undisturbed. No urethral catheter is used. Actually aiding in identification of the urethra and the bladder edge is the partially filled bladder. Two vaginal fingers now aid in cleaning suture sites for precise suture placement and determination of suture sites by pushing lateral vaginal wall against pelvic wall for the proper "fit". One side is completed first, allowing for minor adjustment on the second side, when necessary. The first suture is placed at the posterior urethral level, where it fits against the Tendinous arch, just behind the pubic bone. One or two additional paraurethral and two to five additional paravesical sutures are placed on each side, as indicated by the arrows. After all sutures are placed on one side, the sutures are tied from front to back, while vaginal fingers approximate the tissues to avoid tissue tension during the process.

Below, all sutures have been tied, the urethra now rests comfortably in its new hammock, the posterior urethrovesical angle is now normal and intrapelvic, the lateral vaginal defects have been bridged with firm fascial tissues, and anatomic restoration has been completed.

From E. B. Cantor, Female Urinary Stress Incontinence, 1st Ed., 1979. Courtesy of Charles C Thomas, Springfield, Ill.

the normal grade 0 station. Indeed, suspension of the vaginal cuff at the normal level of the ischial spines is the first step in any anterior and posterior vaginal repair.

Reparative Concepts.   Careful dissection reveals three basic defects found with pelvic support loss—midline, lateral and superior (pre- and post-cervical). Major midline defects require midline fascial plication for repair, lateral defects require reattachment along the LLL and ALL, superior defects require reattachment to cervix or to remaining anterior or posterior vaginal cuff. Midline plication actually places lateral defects under additional stress, as does lateral reattachment stress midline defects. Neither repair corrects superior defects. Since defect combinations are common, one may find it necessary to repair all three types of defects in the same segment, even in the same site. Abdominally, if precervical and midline cystocele defects are present, the anterior vaginal cuff may be ellipsed or wedged to remove excess tissues. This wedge is then closed in epithelial and fascial layers, prior to cuff closure. Shortening the lateral cervical ligaments and suspending the vaginal cuff and vault to the uterosacral and culdesac fascia suspends the vaginal cuff at grade 0 station. Abdominal paravaginal (paraurethrovesical) reattachment (Fig. 3)[2-4,13] follows the cuff management, after closing the peritoneum. The same principles are used transvaginally, on both anterior and posterior vaginal repair. As much smooth vaginal epithelium as can be removed is removed, leaving rugated epithelium for better support. Vaginal paravaginal reattachment is usually done via a midline anterior vaginal incision, although bilateral incisions along the LLL offer some distinct advantages. Figures 4a and b[2-4] show the paraurethral portion of the procedure. Paravesical lateral reattachment simply requires extending the paraurethral reattachment back to the ischial spine on each side. Epithelium is then reattached snugly beneath the fascial reattachment. The goal of such restorative surgery is grade 0 status at each of the six vaginal sites, or a Vaginal Profile of 00—00—00 with a functioning, asymptomatic vaginal canal. Midline fascial plications[8,9] and abdominal symphyseal urethropexy[10] procedures need no special comment.

Review Results

Although Tables 1-4 are self-explanatory, a few comments are warranted here. The average age of 70.5 years of the geriatric group offers maximum contrast for comparison with

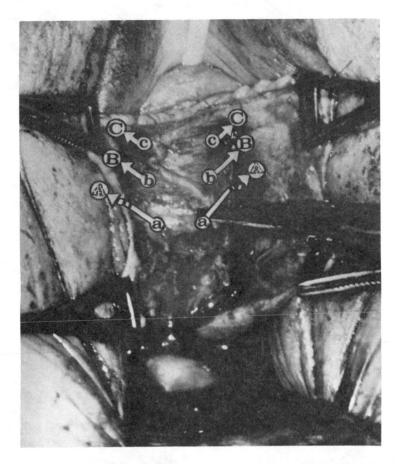

Figure 10:4. Transvaginal Bilateral Paraurethrovesical Reattachment.

a. The technique for the paraurethral portion of the repair with the concepts for completion of the anterior repair. A midline incision of anterior vaginal epithelium has been made, leaving as much fascia on urethra and bladder as possible. Epithelium has been retracted to visualize the anterior, vaginal endopelvic fascial sheath. Obvious urethral and bladder descent to the hymeneal line for an Anterior Vaginal Segment Profile of grade 2 2 is seen. Subpubic urethral rotation and reversal of the posterior Urethrovesical Angle (PUVA) indicate damage to the Pubourethral Ligament Complex (PULC: Posterior, Middle and Anterior). Urethrovesical support loss is virtually always bilateral, with frequent midline, subvesical fascial damage, often associated with pubocervical fascial (precervical) avulsion. Paraurethral reattachment is done by lateral dissection behind the pubic bone, followed by reattachment of posterior paraurethral fascia "a" to the tendinous arch about 1 centimeter behind the pubic bone at "A". Then "b" will be reattached to fascia and remnants of the deep transverse perineal muscle on the same side; "c" may or may not require reattachment in the region of the Anterior Pubourethral Ligament (C). One side is completed first, allowing for minor adjustments on the second side.

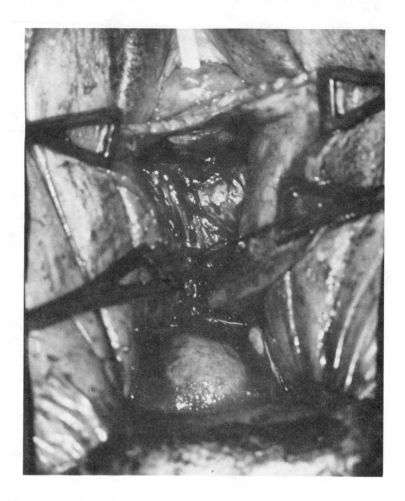

b. The paraurethral reattachment has been completed, leaving the urethra at a grade 0 station. Next, when necessary, superior fascial reattachment to cervix or vaginal cuff is performed. Midline fascial defects are then plicated in the midline. Any remaining lateral defects are then reattached along the tendinous arches from the urethral reattachment area back to ischial spine on either side. Vaginal epithelium is always snugly reattached beneath lateral and superior fascial reattachments. Little, if any, epithelial trimming is required with reattachment procedures. Posterior rectocele defects are similar to, and repaired like, the cystocele defects.

From E. B. Cantor, Female Urinary Stress Incontinence, 1st Ed., 1979. Courtesy of Charles C Thomas, Springfield, Ill.

TABLE 1.   COMPARISON OF PREOPERATIVE DATA.

Data	65+ Group		−40 Group	
Age in years: Range, average	65–83	70.5	24–39	33.7
Parity: Range, average	0–11	2.7	1–5	2.9
Weight (pounds): Range, average	108–186	145.2	104–218	141.6
Prior surgical repair:		5		0
Severity at worst site: Average (grade)	2.9			1.9
Complications: Urinary	4			2
Pulmonary	2			0
Cardiovascular	17			1
Other	4			0
Totals	27			3
Infections: No prophylaxis	4/20	20.0%	9/23	39.1%
With prophylaxis	2/24	8.3%	4/21	19.1%

the −40 group, averaging 33.7 years of age (Table 1). The parity of both groups was surprisingly equal, in view of the modern contraceptive-oriented younger group. Only the 65+ group had survived long enough to require repair of prior operative failures in five patients (11.4%). In a similar vein, the 65+ group had survived long enough, passing through menopausal changes en route, to average severity of grade 2.9 support loss at their worst sites, compared to only 1.9 grade for the −40 group. This indicates the 65+ group had one or more sites with descent half-way past the hymen, while the −40 group descended only to the hymen. By and large the repairs were much more difficult in the 65+ group because of this increased severity. The 65+ group suffered 27 preoperative complications, mostly hypertension, compared to only three in the −40 group. Age does take its toll, yet there was no mortality in either group and all complications responded to the indicated management. Prophylactic antibiotics appear useful, although the −40 group suffered approximately double the infection complications. In the 65+ group, 4 of 20 (20%) of patients without prophylaxis developed infections, while with antibiotics, only two (8.3%) of 24 developed infections. This is in contrast to nine (39.1%) of 23 without antibiotics, and four (19.6%) with antibiotics, in the −40 group.

Table 2 reveals that postoperative complications were comparable, except for a temperature of 101° or more, where the −40 group again exceeded the 65+ group by seven (15.9%) to none. This temperature criterion was used prior to more recent standardization and so was continued. The need for postoperative catheters was 34 (77.3%) in the older group,

TABLE 2. POSTOPERATIVE DATA COMPARISON.

		65+ Group		−40 Group	
Complications:	None	29	65.9%	29	65.9%
	101+ fever	0	0	7	15.9%
	Cellulitis/abscess	2	4.5%	2	4.5%
	Urinary (lower)	10	22.7%	7	15.9%
	Pulmonary	1	2.3%	1	2.3%
	Other	3	6.8%	3	6.8%
	Total	16		20	
Catheter:					
	None required	10	22.7%	21	47.7%
	Required	34	77.3%	23	52.3%
	Days required: Range, average	0–13	2.5	0–10	1.6
Hospital days: Range, average		4–13	5.6	3–11	5.9

compared to only 23 (52.3%) in the younger group. The 65+ group needed a catheter for an average of 2.5 days, compared to only 1.6 days in the −40 group, both figures exceptionally short for reparative procedures. Hospital days following surgery were 5.6 and 5.9, respectively, denoting marked tolerance and resilience in the older group.

Table 3 shows the cure rates for both groups by sites and segments. We do not accept symptomatic relief alone for cure. We further require an asymptomatic, grade 0 or 1 anatomic restoration, a radical departure from standard practice, but one we believe necessary. Many grade 2 defects, for example, are relatively asymptomatic, yet obviously abnormal. In

TABLE 3. REPARATIVE RESULTS BY SITES AND SEGMENTS.*

Sites	Cure			
Segments	65+ Group		−40 Group	
Urethral (Urethrocele)	31/35	88.6%	25/27	92.6%
Bladder (Cystocele)	31/34	91.2%	24/27	88.9%
Anterior Vaginal Segment	32/38	84.2%	29/32	90.6%
Uterine (Prolapse)	33/34	97.1%	38/38	100%
Culdesac (Enterocele)	11/11	100%	22/22	100%
Superior Vaginal Segment	35/36	97.2%	38/38	100%
Rectal (Rectocele)	24/25	96.0%	14/14	100%
Perineal (Chronic laceration)	26/26	100%	16/16	100%
Posterior Vaginal Segment	25/26	96.2%	16/16	100%

*Site cure requires relief of symptoms and anatomic restoration to Grade 0 or 1 status at the site. Segment cure requires cure of both involved sites in a given segment, as stated.

TABLE 4.   RESULTS OF URETHRAL REPAIR BY TECHNIQUE.*

Technique	Cure			
	65+ Group		−40 Group	
Abdominal Paravaginal Repair	10/12	83.3%	15/15	100%
Vaginal Paravaginal Repair	18/20	90.0%	9/11	81.8%
Abdominal Symphyseal Urethropexy				
(MMK)	1/1	100%	0/0	100%
Vaginal Midline Plication	2/2	100%	1/1	100%
Totals	31/35	88.8%	25/27	92.6%

*Cure requires both relief of symptoms (incontinence) and anatomic restoration to Grade 0 or 1 status.
65+ Group: Only one failure in the last 20 patients (95% cure).
−40 Group: Only one failure in the last 22 patients (95.5% cure).

addition, we require that *both* sites in a given segment meet the same criteria for a segmental cure. We fully realize this gives our results a severe handicap when compared to other reports, but it also makes our data more accurate in our view. In Table 3 it is obvious that the anterior vaginal segment remains the chief cause of failures. Yet the average cure rate for all 291 of the total sites operated was 95%. Unpublished data since 1976 (Baden and Walker) reveal a cure rate approximating 95% for the urethra, bladder and the anterior vaginal segment, after we had gained more expertise in identifying and repairing the precise defects. Table 4 points out comparable cure rates for both transvaginal and abdominal routes when utilizing the paravaginal repair techniques. Again, the majority of our failures occurred in the earlier stages of the study. Since 1976, only one failure to relieve urinary incontinence was noted in each group, with 19 (95%) of 20 in the 65+ group and 21 (95.5%) of 22 in the −40 group being cured.

Problems Pitfalls Solutions

1. *Age* per se is not a contraindication to surgery. *Complications* of aging are the problem. The *pitfall* is undertaking surgery without full evaluation and therapy to bring the patient up to her optimal status, preoperatively. Geriatric patients have less resistance to intra- and postoperative complications, which then may rapidly compound. The *solution* is teamwork through liberal consultations.

2. *Prior repair* is not a contraindication. The *pitfall* is difficulty in developing the anatomy necessary for repair.

Bowel or bladder entry is a hazard. The *solution* is to know anatomy, use the abdominal route when necessary in lieu of "blind" posterior colpotomy, place a sound in the bladder or a finger in the rectum for identification and leave as much fascia on both bladder and bowel walls as possible.

3. *Estrogen deficiency* causes thinner tissues with which to work. The *pitfalls* are possible bowel or bladder entry and poor healing. The alternative, preoperative estrogen priming, causes more vascularity, possibly resulting in more blood loss, hematomata and infections. Our *solution* is to give estrogens beginning a day or two after surgery. This avoids excess blood loss, yet quickly provides healthy tissues for proper healing.

4. *Postoperative* complications are a problem. The *pitfall* is delayed therapy and compounding of complications. The *solution* is to keep ahead of potential complications. Prevention is best, early treatment second in importance. We feel antibiotics are valuable allies, prophylactically. Day-of-surgery ambulation and avoidance of routine catheters are helpful.

5. *Increased severity of the defects* is the rule in the older patient. The *pitfall* is edema, thickening, leatherization of the epithelium and loss of tissue planes for proper dissection. The *solution* is preoperative estrogen in these instances, temporary pessary placement to keep the tissues moist inside the hymeneal ring, and extreme care during dissection. The bladder is difficult to free from a small, soft, atrophic uterus. Palpation, aided by a sound in the uterine canal, will be helpful. It is better to dissect into the cervix than the bladder. To prevent these problems, we also recommend repair at the symptomatic, grade 2, or early grade 3 station, prior to major protrusion, if the patient concurs.

6. *Immobility of the hip joints* preventing the lithotomy position needed for repair. The *pitfall* is not realizing that *prolapse of the uterus, enterocele and urethrocystocele are often better managed by the abdominal route*. The *solution*: these patients can usually be completely relieved of superior and anterior vaginal segment support loss, in spite of their immobility. Even rectocele slack may be partially corrected by adequate suspension of the vaginal cuff and vault. Only perineal laceration is totally beyond repair through the abdominal route.

7. *Misdiagnosis* of the defects with incorrect repair as the *pitfall* has been frequent in past years. The *solution*: learn to properly diagnose midline, lateral and superior defects and to

identify them at surgery. Precise repair easily follows and offers optimal cure.

8. *Postoperative sexual activity* is desired by many older women. The *pitfall* is shortening, tunneling, or funneling of the vaginal canal. Shortening is due to failure to elevate the vaginal cuff and vault on the uterosacral and lateral cervical ligaments to a grade 0 station. Tunneling is due to excessive midline fascial plication either anteriorly or posteriorly. One firm fascial plication is adequate for repair of intrinsic defects. Instead of further layers of plication, lateral reattachment of the fascia along the lateral levator lines offers a more anatomic repair with no vaginal narrowing and minimal trimming of vaginal epithelium. Funneling is a combination of both shortening and tunneling. The *solutions* are as described. Remember, too, that these postmenopausal women have dry vaginal tissues. They need an adequate introital opening to compensate for this and for the poor penile erections often found in geriatric men.

9. *Patient reluctance* to undergo repair stems from fear of failure, assuming she is "too old" and many other reasons. The *pitfall* is that without gentle encouragement, she might be condemned to her pitiful existence for the rest of her life. The *solution* for women in relatively good health is frank discussion, perhaps a pessary while she is making up her mind and a daughter, or friend, who has had a successful repair. "Forcing" surgery is entirely wrong, but the correctly informed patient will usually eventually request repair. Many older patients have stated "they would rather be dead than live like this." With current medical advances and reparative techniques, most such patients need not "live like that."

Summary and Conclusions

To evaluate the management, to ascertain the tolerance and to determine the results of elective, reparative procedures in the geriatric female, 44 patients averaging 70.5 years of age were matched with 44 women averaging 33.7 years of age. Functional pelvic supportive anatomy was stressed. Support loss severity was evaluated by grading each of the six vaginal sites from 0–4, using the Half-way Grading System. The types of defects found were traditional midline fascial, lateral (paravaginal) and superior (pre- and postcervical) in location. Differentiation of the three defect types was accomplished by observations made during the straining descent (HWGS) and during holding (pubococcygeal contraction) ascent or lack of

154

ascent. This permits preoperative defect diagnosis and true individualization of therapy. When the defects are confirmed at operation, they are repaired by the specific techniques indicated for each defect type. These techniques are midline fascial plication for midline defects, lateral (paravaginal) reattachment for lateral defects, and superior reattachment for pre- and postcervical defects. Since the defects tend to be multiple, it is often necessary to blend the reparative techniques together, often at a single site. Postoperative status was compared to the preoperative defects at six weeks, six months and then annually, following the surgery. Both relief of symptoms and anatomic restoration are required for a cure at each site. Both sites in a given segment must be cured for cure of the segment. The need for these strict requirements was stressed; and problems causing pitfalls and the solutions were discussed.

There was no mortality in the population studied, and the morbidity was acceptable in both groups. Prophylactic antibiotics did seem to offer some protection from the infectious complications. The 65+ group required postoperative catheter use in 77.3% for an average of 2.5 days, with the average hospital stay of 5.6 days. This compared to catheter use in 52.3% for an average of 1.6 days and with a hospital stay of 5.9 days in the −40 group. Of the total 291 vaginal sites operated, only 14 (4.8%) failures occurred in both groups, one at six weeks, one at six months, 11 at one year and one at two years, postoperatively. Failure rates were 5.5% and 3.9% for the 65+ and −40 groups, respectively. Of the 186 segments operated in both groups, the failure rate was 5.9%, with comparable figures in each group. The anterior vaginal segment remains the enigma, with 84.2% to 90.6% cure for the 65+ and −40 groups. In recent years, both groups have risen to 95% cure in this segment and for relief of urinary incontinence.

Conclusions From the Study are:

1. With meticulous preoperative, intraoperative and postoperative management, virtually all geriatric women can be prepared for these elective, reparatory procedures, will tolerate them well and obtain the same excellent results as their younger sisters.

2. Adequate knowledge of functional supportive anatomy will permit preoperative diagnosis of the defect types and planning of true individualized therapy. Operative confirma-

tion of the defects and precise repair by the specific technique for each defect type will then assure optimal cure.

3. Multiple sites, segments and defect types are the rule. A blend of traditional midline fascial plication with lateral and superior reattachment techniques should achieve 95% cure rates, even in the elderly patient with severe support loss and in spite of the stricter definition for cure.

4. Problems and pitfalls involved in the management of the geriatric patients are largely avoidable or correctable.

5. On the basis of this study, the geriatric female with pelvic support loss should be encouraged to request vaginal reparative procedures for an improved quality of life, just as are young patients.

REFERENCES

1. Baden WF, Walker T. Genesis of the vaginal profile. Clin Obstet Gynecol 15:1048-1054, 1972.
2. Baden WF, Walker T. Evaluation of the stress incontinent patient. *In* Cantor EB (ed.). Female Urinary Stress Incontinence, 1st ed. Springfield, Charles C Thomas, 1979, pp. 142-148.
3. *Ibid.*, pp. 157-158.
4. *Ibid.*, pp. 172-174.
5. Baden WF, Walker T, Lindsey JH. The vaginal profile. Tex Med 64: 56-58, 1968.
6. Harbrecht PJ, Garrison RN, Fry DE. Surgery in the elderly patient. South Med J 74:594-598, 1981.
7. Kegel AH. The nonsurgical treatment of genital relaxation. Ann West Med Surg 2:213-216, 1948.
8. Kelly HA. Incontinence of urine in women. Urol cutan Rev 17:291-293, 1913.
9. Kennedy WT. Urinary incontinence relieved by restoration and maintenance of normal position of urethra. Am J Obstet Gynecol 41:16-28, 1941.
10. Marshall VF, Marchetti AA, Krantz KF. The correction of stress by simple vesicourethral suspension. Surg Gynecol Obstet 88:509-518, 1949.
11. Milley PS, Nichols DH. The relationship between the pubourethral ligaments and the urogenital diaphragm in the human female. Anat Rec 170:281-283, 1971.
12. Nichols DH. Retrorectal levatorplasty with colporrhaphy. Clin Obstet Gynecol 25:939-947, 1982.
13. Richardson AC, Edmonds PB, Williams NL. Treatment of stress urinary incontinence due to paravaginal fascial defects. Obstet Gynecol 57:357-362, 1981.
14. Sourcebook on Aging 1st ed. Chicago, Marquis Academic Media, Who's Who Inc., 1977.

15. Stanton SL, Tanagho EA. Preface. *In* Stanton SL, Tanagho EA (eds.). Surgery of Female Incontinence (1st ed.). New York, Springer-Verlag, 1980.
16. Tancer ML. Geriatric gynecologic surgery. OB-Gyn Digest:41–52, 1968.
17. United States Bureau of Census. Statistical Abstracts of the United States, 1981, Tables 29, 30.
18. White GR. An anatomic operation for cure of cystocele. Am J Obst Dis Wom Child 65:286–290, 1912.

11

MANAGING PROLAPSE OF THE POST-HYSTERECTOMY VAGINA

JESSE A. RUST, M.D.

Management of inversion (eversion or turning inside out) of the post-hysterectomy vagina has long been an enigma for the gynecologic surgeon, as evidenced by the number and variety of corrective procedures that have evolved. With the increasing numbers of abdominal and vaginal hysterectomies now being performed on our younger female population, it seems inevitable that the incidence of prolapse of the vaginal vault will certainly increase. It would behoove the gynecologic surgeon in training today to take advantage of every opportunity to observe or participate in the correction of this condition. Almost always the vagina, as a functioning structure, should be maintained. The Sex Information and Education Council of the United States and the National Institute on Aging have indicated that most people may continue to enjoy sexual relations throughout their lifetime, even though a patient may profess absolute lack of interest in participating in future sexual activity. The ability to do so should be preserved if at all possible. Certainly with our geriatric population increasing in numbers and longevity, and with improved general health, efforts to preserve sexual function become increasingly more important.

The etiology of prolapse of the uterus is somewhat different from that of prolapse of a post-hysterectomy vaginal vault. Prolapse of the uterus no doubt results from an inherent weakness of the ligaments and fascial supporting structures that have become attenuated and of poor quality. Poor obstetrical care has been blamed and is no doubt partially responsible for prolapse of the uterus, whereas poor surgical attention to this problem leads to later prolapse of the vaginal vault. Special attention to the uterosacral and cardinal ligaments and to the occult enterocele (deep posterior cul-de-sac) and repair of the pelvic floor are essential. A simple perineorrhaphy is not adequate in most instances.

In recent years it has become generally accepted that vaginal hysterectomy and repair of pelvic floor relaxation have rightly replaced, in most instances, the surgical procedures that were popular a generation or so ago. The Manchester–Fothergill operation, the Watkins transposition operation, and the partial obliterative procedures on the vagina even today may have rare indications. It would behoove the gynecologic surgeon to continue to be familiar with these procedures and their indications, although he will very rarely be called upon to do any of them.

The Manchester–Fothergill operation is still an occasionally useful procedure as in, for example, the relatively young career woman who has the unfortunate experience of prolapse of the uterus following a pregnancy early in her reproductive years. This operation can usually be accomplished without amputation of the cervix unless it is markedly elongated and protruding through the introitus (amputation of the cervix will no doubt make the cervix incompetent and a successful pregnancy questionable), and if done properly, will leave the patient able to reproduce if her desires change and pregnancy becomes important. If this operation has been successfully accomplished and pregnancy does occur, a cesarean section would most likely be indicated. The operation may be offered to the woman who refuses, in spite of adequate information, to allow the removal of a normal uterus. The Watkins interposition or transposition operation is probably less important, but it is easily performed when the cervix does not protrude much beyond the introitus and when there is a huge cystocele with very thinned out vesicovaginal fascia on an elderly woman in poor general health. Incidentally, we removed the uterus in one patient on whom this had been performed and found the vaginal removal of the transposed uterus not a difficult procedure (a diagnostic D&C had been performed beforehand). The partial colpocleisis is probably rarely, if ever, indicated today, since it results in a retained uterus that is inaccessible if bleeding problems occur.

When abdominal hysterectomy is indicated, it is extremely important that the pelvic relaxation should be evaluated and, if possible, corrected at the same time as the hysterectomy is performed. If not, the patient should have regular follow-up examinations, and with evidence of increased relaxation and vaginal protrusion, repair should be recommended before complete prolapse of the vagina occurs. At abdominal hysterectomy, the uterosacral ligaments can easily be identified with traction on the uterus or on the top of the vagina after the uterus has been removed. The cul-de-sac peritoneum can be excised back to the bowel quite easily with blunt dissection, and the uterosacral ligaments plicated with figure-of-eight sutures.

The diagnosis of prolapse of the vaginal vault with the vagina completely turned inside out is not difficult. However, when the patient reports "My bladder is falling out," it behooves the gynecologist to evaluate the problem very carefully. The situation may present a prolapsed vault, a huge cystocele, or huge rectoenterocele, or all three. The single blade of a bivalved speculum holding the anterior wall up should easily identify posterior wall relaxations. The blade turned over and held downward will permit demonstration of a cystocele, and by identifying scar tissue and applying gentle traction with an Allis clamp, the examiner can confirm the presence of a prolapse of the vaginal vault.

Treatment of post-hysterectomy prolapse of the vaginal vault falls into three general areas:

1. Pessary—Gellhorn or doughnut
2. Vaginal operations
    A. Anterior and posterior colporrhaphy, at which time enterocele peritoneum is excised and uterosacral and cardinal ligaments identified and approximated. Extensive repair of the vesicovaginal and rectovaginal fascia and perineal body
    B. Colpocleisis, complete
    C. Colpocleisis, partial
        1) Extensive anterior and posterior repair with a high perineal body, leaving a douche-tip caliber vagina
        2) The LeFort procedure
        3) Suture of the vaginal vault to the right sacrospinous ligament
3. Abdominal operations
    A. Sacral colpopexy with polyester mesh (Mersilene or Propolene) is listed first in this category, because it has been our procedure of choice for over 10 years and has produced gratifying results. All other abdominal approaches pull the vault forward and expose the cul-de-sac to enterocele development
    B. Vault sutured to the anterior abdominal wall
    C. Use of homologous tissue strips
        1) Fascia lata
            a) Anterior rectus fascia
            b) Extraperitoneal or cross-suspended behind the bladder

2) Dermal graft
3) Cooper's ligaments
D. Collagen mesh in which the vaginal vault is wrapped with collagen to reinforce the remaining ligamentous structures has been suggested.

We classify post-hysterectomy prolapse of the vaginal vault into two types, depending basically on the caliber of the vagina after the prolapse has been replaced by the examining fingers.

Type I—Large caliber with cystocele, rectocele, lacerated perineum and almost always enterocele. Best repaired vaginally.

Type II—Small or normal caliber vagina. Best repaired abdominally.

There are patients whose prolapse falls somewhere between the two types. For example: one with a high perineal body and cystocele or enterocele; better repaired vaginally after episiotomy.

Marshall-Marchetti-Krantz type of operation may be performed safely with either type. No vaginal repair should be done at the same time as the abdominal if foreign material, such as Mersilene mesh, is used, because the danger of infection could be serious and necessitate removal of the mesh.

If repair of Type II prolapse is accomplished vaginally, the vagina is almost always sacrificed as a functioning structure.

Repair of Type I Prolapse

The repair of Type I is, of course, much the same as that for the prolapsed uterus. The scar tissue where the cervix was removed can usually be identified, and with traction on it and dissection, the cul-de-sac peritoneum is easily found and should be removed back to its reflection from the bowel.

With traction on each side, close to the aforementioned scar tissue, bands of endopelvic fascia can almost always be identified extending laterally and posteriorly; these are no doubt attenuated uterosacral ligaments with cardinal ligament tissue above. After excision of the cul-de-sac peritoneum, these ligaments should be plicated back as far as possible toward the bowel, and the distal end of the approximated ligamentous tissue sutured under the cystocele repair. Repair of the cystocele is done as usual, and repair of the rectocele and perineal body is done through a double Diamond (Emmet) denudation. In repairing the rectocele we start suturing the mucous membrane first with a continuous lock-stitch suture of 0 chromic catgut. After it has been approximated down toward the introitus 4 to 5 cm, a Sims speculum is inserted beneath the mucous membrane, elevating it and pushing it back in. Then the rectovaginal fascia is plicated with interrupted figure-of-eight sutures in two or more layers. This creates depth to the post repair and eliminates "dashboard" perineum. As these layers are brought down toward the perineal body, the closure of the mucous membrane is advanced in stages with a continuous lock-stitch suture. Levator fascia, if identifiable, may be approximated without taking huge, deep bites which cause postoperative pain and are of perhaps little lasting value. The perineal body is built up with interrupted figure-of-eight sutures. When brought to the hymenal level, a loop of the mucous membrane suture is held and continued downward toward the anus subcutaneously, then back up subcuticularly and tied to the loop near the hymenal level. Utilization of a Sims speculum as the posterior repair progresses is suggested, particularly to get depth to the pelvic floor, which is so markedly relaxed in these patients. With informed consent, the patient is told that (when the vaginal approach is taken) at some future date a recurrence is always possible and, at that time, will possibly necessitate an abdominal operation.

Repair of Type II Prolapse

For Type II prolapse, we have selected the same procedure for about 12 years, colpopexy with Mersilene mesh to the presacral tissues. We have one special instrument, which is nothing more than a curved ring forceps bent to nearly a right angle about halfway between the hinge and the distal part that holds the sponge. With the patient in position with the knees spread and supported as for retropubic urinary stress incontinence, the sponge forceps carrying a tightly folded 4 × 4 gauze sponge, well lubricated, is inserted into the vagina to elevate the vault upward toward the abdominal incision, which will be a Pfannenstiel type. With the bladder emptied and continuous catheter drainage, the abdomen is opened and the knob of the vaginal vault is easily accessible. The peritoneum is stripped down posteriorly from it as far as can be reached. An incision is made through the peritoneum over the anterior surface of the sacrum from near the promontory downward about 6 or 8 cm, and the peritoneum is then loosened down under the cul-de-sac quite easily by blunt dissection with a finger. A double-thick strip of Mersilene mesh, about the width of the vaginal vault and about 10 to 12 cm long, has been prepared. A kidney pedicle clamp (i.e. a question-mark type of clamp, not a right-angle clamp) is then inserted in the incision over the sacrum and, by further blunt dissection, is carried under the peritoneum to the denuded area posterior to the knob of the vagina, keeping to the right of the bowel. The Mersilene mesh has been attached to the vaginal knob with 6 or 8 very fine sutures of synthetic No. 3 Teflon or other similar material, taking extreme care not to perforate the vaginal mucous membrane. The free end of the mesh is then pulled under the peritoneum and attached to the periosteum anterior to the sacrum, usually at about the level of the second sacral vertebra. Three figure-of-eight sutures are used; Surgilon 0 is our preference, the suture especially prepared for retropubic urethro-vesical suspension. After attaching the Mersilene mesh to the sacrum, the excess is cut away. In pulling the mesh beneath the peritoneum, it is not always possible to have it retroperitoneal all the way when the pelvis is very deep, the bowel voluminous, and the patient obese, in which case the peritoneum may be opened exposing the mesh part of the way. The peritoneum in this area is so bunched up that the tape is not visible in the peritoneal cavity. The sigmoid colon could be sutured over this, but this measure is probably unnecessary. When attached to the sacrum, the Mersilene mesh should not be pulled too tightly, because straightening the anterior vaginal wall might contribute to stress urinary incontinence. The peritoneum over the sacrum and over the vaginal knob is then closed, and the abdomen closed in the usual manner.

Sacral colpopexy is a relatively simple, though major, surgical procedure. One needs to be familiar with pelvic anatomy and to operate carefully, especially avoiding penetration of the vagina, the middle sacral vessels and, of course, the ureters. Staying close to the cul-de-sac peritoneum has avoided any bleeding deep in the pelvis. At present it is the preferred operation for Type II eversion of the vagina.

12

CARE OF THE DYING PATIENT

JAMES L. BREEN, M.D.
ALBERT STRUNK, M.D., J.D.

To some extent death and dying, as a topic, has become a fad. Much of the current writing leaves one under the impression that society has determined that previously accepted modes and circumstances of death are inappropriate and often distasteful. Moreover, one senses an implicit notion that, as a society, we have discovered the right way to die—"death with dignity"—and what is left to be done is to require the medical profession to implement these new truths and methods in caring for patients so that we may feel the same sense of well-being and satisfaction in the management of death as we do in the management of birth. Indeed the work of Kubler-Ross has had effects surely not envisioned by its author wherein patients have been marched through the Five Stages of Dying to their "acceptance" of imminent death with a vigorousness worthy of military drill.

We do not make this observation with any sense that our own approach to the dying patient is superior to that of anyone else, or that our own suggestions may not be misconstrued and misapplied. Rather, the observation is made to underline the point that there is no "method" or generalized schema applicable in the care and treatment of dying patients. Here, as in the practice of medicine as a whole, the appropriateness of any regimen which is undertaken must be measured in regard to the needs of the individual patient. To insure that the patient's individualized needs are met requires that the privacy of the physician-patient relationship be maintained against the well-intentioned but frequently misguided importunities of family and friends, administrators, sometimes lawyers and judges, and society at large.

General Considerations

The process of dying is progressive and not really a simultaneous failure of all vital functions. In speaking of care of the dying, we should realize that according to the oldest adage, the process usually starts from below upwards. The sensation and power of motion, as well as reflexes, are lost in the legs before the arms; and in the intestinal tract the anal sphincters relax, peristalsis ceases, and the stomach distends, before the patient can no longer swallow. Under such conditions, the folly of attempting to give medicines by mouth is apparent, for it will be regurgitated; so here we get into intravenous fluids and hyperalimentation, if there is hope for rejuvenation and some degree of "worthwhile" survival. The absurdity of forcing fluids becomes even more glaring when such fluids enter the trachea and give forth an "iatrogenic" death rattle.

As long as the patient can swallow, fluids should be given. Except for the drawing in of the breath, sucking is the body's *last*, as it is the *first*, instinctive action. Thirst is our first and last craving. The complaint just before death on the cross was *I thirst*.

Although the patient's mouth is generally open in the last hours, we must not forget the biblical phrase of the "tongue cleaving to the top of the mouth." Tremendous misery may result from the lack of saliva in a terminal phase, but nurses can prevent this by applying bits of ice enmeshed in gauze, or adding vaseline to the tongue. It is interesting that when ice is placed in gauze, its moisture evaporates without bringing about the tracheal ingestion of fluid. On the other hand, we fear aspiration by patients where there is too much fluid in the mouth. In such situations, the patient should be turned on her side to allow for gravity drainage.

We should realize that just simple change in posture often relieves the dying patient's general discomfort. When patients are in extremis, or unconscious, and are found lying flat on their back, it is because they are not able to make known their need for help or to shift themselves from that position; they may still appreciate the comfort that a change affords, nevertheless.

When respiration is labored, "dilating" the upper half of the thorax is beneficial, i.e., as Florence Nightingale pointed out in her notes on nursing, it is important to pillow the head so that the neck shall not flex on the body and thus allow better oxygenation. As peripheral circulation diminishes, there is usually an increased amount of perspiration. The body's surface cools regardless of the temperature of the room. It is important, therefore, to sponge the patient, to change linens often. Bladder distention, which we so often overlook, may require urinary drainage.

In addition, the patient's hospital area should be well

illuminated, for "the chamber should be well lighted as the patient enters the valley of the shadows." Dying patients, as long as they are able to, instinctively turn toward light. Some will even complain of growing darkness. As sight and hearing diminish, the dying see only what is near and hear only what is distinctly spoken to them. I think the most imperative thing we as physicians must do is to be present and to give the final support, whether it is to touch, hold a hand, or take a pulse. It has been stated that many enjoy soothing music, and in the Feierabendhaus of the Deaconess Hospital in Germany, where the dying are more beautifully cared for than anywhere else in the world, hymns are played for them on the organ in the adjoining chapel.

A Continuum of Care

A distinction is made by some authors between treatment for palliation and treatment for cure. In approaching the care of a terminal patient this dichotomy should be avoided for several reasons. First, it is rarely possible to neatly divide treatment modalities into purely therapeutic or curative endeavors on one hand and purely palliative, supportive or maintenance endeavors on the other. Second, even in those instances offering no hope of cure, an aggressive therapeutic regimen may offer some prospect for remission or at least a slowing of the disease process. Third, a perspective about care and treatment demonstrably suitable in approaching a terminal patient with non-malignant disease may not be entirely appropriate for the terminal patient with malignant disease. Fourth, just as our ability to prospectively assess the response of the patient to any therapeutic regimen is limited, even more imperfect is our ability to know when death may ensue in irreparable and irreversible illness.

Mention of these considerations simply emphasizes that there is a continuum of care which must be afforded the terminal patient. This continuum will include intervention directed toward cure of the fundamental pathologic process, possible remission of the pathologic process or a slowing of its progress, the elimination or containment of secondary or superimposed pathologic processes, relief of suffering and maintenance of the patient's physical and emotional comfort and, finally, care of the body and maintenance of vital body and organ functions when the sensorium (consciousness or mental clarity) has been lost. At St. Christopher's Hospice in

London, it is interesting to note that the continuum of care extends to the cleansing of a deceased patient's body and preparation of her remains by those who cared for her while she was alive.

While we alluded, by way of distinction, to the dying patient with non-malignant disease, it is not our intention to discuss such patients here. The specific treatment of end-stage cardiovascular, pulmonary, renal, hepatic or other disease, as well as massive trauma or obstetric hemorrhage is not the subject of this chapter. Our concern is with the patient who is dying from malignant disease of the female reproductive system; as a practical matter these are patients with terminal illnesses secondary to malignancies of the vulva, vagina, cervix, uterus, Fallopian tubes and ovaries, as well as gestational trophoblastic disease.

Some of the specific problems encountered in patients dying from gynecologic malignancies include acute hemorrhage, chronic anemia of malignant disease, immunosuppression secondary to chemotherapy and radiotherapy, uremia, bowel obstruction, ascites, as well as dehydration and electrolyte imbalance. The most pressing problem is, of course, the relief of intolerable, unremitting pain.

Pain and Analgesia

Good nursing care and the relief of pain are, when all is said and done, the two most important features in the care of the dying patient. Concepts adopted concerning the use of analgesia in relationship to postoperative patients or patients with types of disease other than terminal malignancies are inappropriate at best and unspeakably cruel at worst if they limit the appropriate use of analgesics. Clearly there is no place for vaunted concern about drug dependence or drug addiction in a patient whose maximal life expectancy is measured in days or weeks. Yet such concerns emerge repeatedly by way of explanation or justification as one inquires why a patient failed to receive a dose of narcotics required by a standing order. Admittedly, resistance to dispensing narcotic analgesics as ordered is most often encountered in the nurse or physician newly arrived on the oncology service, but vestiges of this resistance are manifested among those physicians whose terminal patients consistently receive slightly less narcotic than they need to be comfortable, rather than slightly more.

Pain may be relieved by several modalities including narcotic or non-narcotic medications, surgery, anesthesia, acupuncture and nerve stimulators. Narcotic and non-narcotic medications, whether administered by mouth, vein, or by subcutaneous or intramuscular injection, are the most common agents utilized. The so-called Brompton's cocktail, popularized at St. Christopher's Hospice, is an excellent oral agent for pain relief. Also available in pre-mixed preparations are morphine elixirs or suspensions which contain up to 20 mg morphine sulfate per teaspoon. We have found the latter to be particularly useful for patients at home.

Once a patient is hospitalized, particularly for the last hospitalization, our preference has been for intravenous morphine sulfate delivered via some type of continuous infusion pump. We are wary of administering these drugs in intravenous infusions without fixed rate pumps simply because of the danger of inadvertent overdosage. These patients usually have peripheral intravenous lines and they are often so cachectic as to make intramuscular injection of analgesia inhumane. Our initial goal is always to achieve complete freedom from pain. We use whatever dosage of morphine is required. Usually this will be 48–96 mg/24 hours. In one patient, we approached 2000 mg/24 hours before pain was abolished. Interestingly, that patient was subsequently weaned completely from intravenous analgesics and lived at home for two additional months on oral and injectable agents before her final hospital admission.

Once pain has been abolished, it is usually possible to progressively diminish the intravenous medication. Progressive diminution of IV meds and substitution with oral and injectable agents becomes our second goal for patients who may possibly be discharged to the home. Obviously this goal need not be pursued for those patients who will never leave the hospital. Commonly employed injectable medications, apart from morphine sulfate, include demerol (Meperidine), Levo-Dromoran (Levorphanol), and Talwin (Pentazocine). It has also been of benefit to use in addition a minor tranquilizer, e.g., Elavil, a major tranquilizer, e.g., Haldol, or a combination psychotropic, e.g., Triavil, to obtain relief of pain. The role of anxiety in heightening the sensation of pain is well appreciated.

One possibility for improved management of analgesia in these patients at home is the use of a continuous subcutaneous injection of opiate and an antiemetic or psychotropic agent via a portable battery-operated infusion pump. Such devices have been used in England with excellent results. Various combinations of opiates, antiemetics and tranquilizers are employed. A butterfly catheter is inserted subcutaneously in the skin of the abdominal wall or in the suprascapular region. The site is changed every 4 to 7 days. The continuous infusion pump, which is worn in a small shoulder holster, delivers its contents over a 24 to 25-hour period. Complications are reportedly few and minor in nature.

In selected cases continuous epidural infusion of morphine may be undertaken. Although this usually means that the patient will not be leaving the hospital, patients have been sent home with such catheters left *in situ*. Although there is an increased risk of infection associated with insertion of an epidural catheter, multiple intramuscular injections are equally or even more likely to cause abscesses at injection sites. Tolerance to analgesia may become a problem but can usually be dealt with by increasing dosage.

Implanted dorsal nerve column stimulators and transcutaneous nerve stimulators also offer a means of dealing with intractable pain. The transcutaneous stimulators provide an adjustable pulsed current source; one such device is adjustable from 0–76 milliamps measured into a 500 OHM load with voltage limited to a maximum of 100 volts. Use of transcutaneous nerve stimulators in a variety of disorders including postoperative pain, pain of malignancy, neuritis and herpes zoster, as well as in the treatment of multiple sclerosis, has been reported.

While it is true that high doses of narcotic or other drugs may hasten a patient's demise (often via respiratory depression, atelectasis, and pneumonia), we remain steadfast in our determination to rid the patient of pain. Any physician or nurse who has any experience caring for patients with terminal malignancies will attest to the extraordinary change in personality and outlook which ensues when the patient is at last relieved of her consuming pain. She is a new person, often with a now acute awareness of her surroundings and a particular interest in communicating with family and friends. We have yet to encounter the patient who chooses to live with pain in order to avoid the use of analgesics.

Hemorrhage

Management of pelvic hemorrhage is usually difficult; it is all the more so in the dying patient. Once effective therapy is no longer available for a cancer patient, primary emphasis is shifted toward management of symptoms, emotional support and avoidance of pain. What is hoped for is a death free of pain, fear and unnecessary stress. When such a patient presents, usually with a persistent or recurrent cervical lesion, management is attempted using packing cryotherapy, cautery, and ligature per vagina. If these modes of treatment are unsuccessful and the patient's overall condition is such as to suggest some added life expectancy were the hemorrhage controlled, arterial embolization is recommended. Such a procedure, usually involving percutaneous puncture through femoral or axillary arteries under local anesthesia, offers minimal morbidity and rare mortality with the prospect of a dramatic solution to a difficult problem.

It is not our intention here to detail the techniques employed in embolization of bleeding pelvic vessels using transarterial pre-shaped catheters introduced via Seldinger puncture. We do wish, nevertheless, to make several points. First, embolization may be appropriately employed even in the absence of a radiographically visible hemorrhage. This is true both with respect to anatomic sources of blood supply and neovascularization. Second, although the technique is most impressive in the context of the acute bleed, chronic bleeding is also susceptible to treatment in this manner. Third, because of the extensive pelvic vascular anastomoses, previous hypogastric ligation is not a bar to use of this technique. Fourth, complications are infrequent but when they do occur, they often involve thrombosis of the vessel through which the catheter has been passed. Obviously, the axillary approach places the renal arteries and branches of the celiac axis at greater risk. Finally, arterial embolization may have some utility for control of pain in selected patients.

Dehydration and electrolyte imbalance

In our experience severe dehydration, with or without electrolyte imbalance, is most often encountered in connection with bowel obstruction, radiation-associated enteritis, or viral syndromes involving the gastrointestinal tract. Immediate admission to the hospital and vigorous intravenous hydration is begun. Naturally hydration must be appropriately adjusted in patients with a history of cardiac disease. If there is a severe electrolyte imbalance, intravenous supplementation is made to correct deficits. The objective is to return the patient to her home at the earliest possible time, even if it appears that readmission will likely be required in the near future. One occasionally hears resident physicians refer to the patient who died in perfect electrolyte balance as though a major treatment goal had been met. To the contrary, in dealing with patients who have terminal malignant disease, it is our intention to afford them as much time as possible outside of the hospital. Once a minimally acceptable level of correction has been achieved via the intravenous route, the patient is returned to a diet, with oral supplementation of electrolytes if needed. Depending on the severity of the patient's condition on admission and the presence or absence of complicating factors (e.g., bowel obstruction), the patient may be discharged even without awaiting a 24 to 48-hour observation period of oral intake.

Bowel Obstruction

Bowel obstruction is frequently encountered in the terminal stages of ovarian carcinoma and, to a lesser extent, cervical carcinoma. Often there are numerous recurrent episodes of partial small bowel obstruction prior to the development of a complete block. Such obstruction may be related to the carcinoma itself, removal of the omentum, radiation therapy, and/or chemotherapy. It may be mechanical, neurogenic or both. The patient is immediately placed on an NPO regimen. Some obstructions will relieve themselves spontaneously simply by placing the bowel at rest. Intravenous fluids are started. Radiographic determination of the level of obstruction is necessary. Where large bowel involvement is found and nonsurgical efforts to relieve the obstruction, such as rectal tubes and high retention enemas, have failed, transverse loop colostomy or even ileostomy may be necessary.

Obstruction of the small bowel is more threatening to the patient's life. Surgical resection of the small bowel is, more often than not, impracticable. Decompression of the stomach and small bowel with Anderson, Miller-Abbot, Cantor or comparable long tubes is the first step. Decadron 10 mg, IV, t.i.d. or q.i.d. has been used empirically to diminish the inflammatory response with mixed results. Nonetheless, use of a steroid is recommended, unless obvious contraindications to steroid therapy exist. Often patients respond to these elementary measures, and the obstruction disappears as evidenced both by the relief of symptoms and follow-up x-ray films. Some patients are able to resume unrestricted diets; most find that bland and soft diets are better tolerated. As tumor involvement with the bowel becomes greater, if is often necessary to discharge patients on liquid diets. While it is recognized that such regimens are often nutritionally inadequate, it is again our objective to minimize the time away from family, friends and familiar surroundings. There is no reason to believe that, except for hyperalimentation (about which more will be said later), the patient's nutrition will be better in the hospital than at home; the reverse is more often true.

In the patient who is in the final stages of her disease with complete, unremitting bowel obstruction and no hope for surgical relief, a breach of the normal protocol concerning NPO regimens while nasogastric or intestinal tubes are *in situ* is appropriate. Our practice is to allow such patients any liquid or solid food by mouth so long as the particle size is sufficiently small to pass the pores of the tube. While it may seem ridiculous to allow a patient to eat what we promptly suck out of her stomach, the benefit to the patient's morale from allowing food to be taken by mouth has been more than enough to justify our departure from orthodox methods. It should be emphasized, however, that we reserve such methods for those who have begun the rapid catabolic decline of complete intractable obstruction and who are only weeks, if not days, from death.

Reference has been made to the use of x-ray studies, notably the obstructive series, in the diagnosis of bowel obstruction. It should be remembered that while such x-ray series are particularly useful during the initial obstructive episodes, there may be little or no utility in obtaining such films of the patient who presents for one of many admissions with recurrent obstruction. The question of whether the radiographic result will modify the treatment to be undertaken must always be asked. Often, in cases of recurrent obstruction where surgical approaches have been ruled out, there will be no point in documenting by x-ray examination a partial or complete obstruction which is diagnosable on clinical examination.

Hyperalimentation

Once the patient with a terminal gynecologic malignancy has become totally bedridden and is no longer able to take food or even water by mouth, death is obviously imminent. The question invariably arises when such a patient is admitted to the hospital whether or not intravenous fluids and, in some cases, hyperalimentation should be started. It is the policy of some institutions not to start intravenous infusions, even of dextrose and water, on such patients where no significant delay in the process of dying can be achieved. In general, hospices do not employ intravenous infusions in this circumstance even for hydration, let alone for supplying calories.

It is usually our practice to initiate hydration via the intravenous route on any dehydrated patient, even if death appears imminent. More often than not such patients rally briefly, regain their lucidity, and have a few days, sometimes weeks, of additional time. Often this is a period in which relationships are reaffirmed and partings exchanged. On the other hand, it has not been our practice to use hyperalimentation with the patient in the terminal phase of her illness. Again this assumes that there is no medical or surgical condition which, if the patient's nutritional status were improved, could be treated.

Ascites and Paracentesis

Treatment of recurrent ascites secondary to malignant gynecologic disease, especially ovarian carcinoma, is a frequently encountered problem. Rather than use vacuum bottles or other suction devices, our approach is to utilize a Dow cystocatheter kit connected to a closed gravity drainage system. If the puncture site has been carefully selected and the patency of the indwelling catheter established, such a tap drains 4 to 8 liters of ascitic fluid in 24 hours, with larger amounts withdrawn from patients who roll from side to side or otherwise move about to mobilize fluid collections toward the area of drainage. Ultrasound scan of the abdomen is useful for localizing fluid pockets, avoiding tumor-studded parietal peritoneum, and ascertaining the existence of abdominal wall adhesions and the proximity of bowel. If paracentesis can be performed under ultrasonographic direction, the margin of safety for avoiding bowel or other organs is increased, but we do not insist on this technique. We customarily perform paracentesis in the patient's hospital room after a careful physical examination. Although we may scan the patient with recurrent malignant ascites from time to time, we do not do so unless the clinical exam presents ambiguous findings which would justify the added cost.

Paracentesis will usually be performed on multiple occasions before the patient dies. Unfortunately, continued successful drainage of large quantities of ascitic fluid is hampered by loculation of fluid and an ever-increasing rate of fluid formation. Taps are not customarily performed until the patient begins to suffer some respiratory embarrassment or intolerable pain. It is our desire to tap the patient as infrequently as possible and to maximize the yield from each tap.

Apart from the obvious desire to tap into a fluid pocket and to avoid bowel, the likelihood of seeding the tract created by the puncture with malignant cells should also be considered. Certainly one should not puncture through a tumor mass of the parietal peritoneum if possible. Apart from that, however, anterior and lateral sites have advantages and disadvantages. The lateral tap will allow better access to the abdominal gutters and afford drainage of more fluid from the patient who usually lies in the dorsosupine position. However, there may be an increased amount of seeding due to the volume of cellular debris which collects in the gutters. Anterior puncture sites are likely to have less seeding, but often do not drain as well. Midline taps will naturally afford the most protection against inadvertent perforation of a vessel.

Chronic Anemia of Malignant Disease

As a result of both radiation therapy and chemotherapy all of the cellular constituents of blood are decreased secondary to both diminished hematopoesis and increased rate of cellular destruction. No fixed rules can be made as to when transfusion of packed red blood cells or other blood components should be given. Clearly the patient who is hemorrhaging secondary to tumor invasion of a vascular bed is not a candidate for continuous blood transfusion if hemostasis cannot be obtained. On the other hand, query whether or not a patient who requires two units of packed cells each month to maintain a minimal oxygen-carrying capacity should be denied such transfusions? In general we have provided blood replacement in such instances with a resultant prolongation of life of 6 to 12 months and occasionally more. Whether or not this is a reasonable expenditure of limited blood resources is debatable and will, of course, be influenced by the supply of blood available at any given time. The use of fresh frozen plasma, platelets and other blood constituents is usually avoided.

Immune Suppression and Antibiotic Treatment

Immune suppression, or incompetence apart from its likely

role in the etiology of malignant disease, is an unfortunate side effect of both chemotherapy and radiotherapy. As indicated in the previous section, it is not our practice to transfuse our dying patients with blood components, including transfusions for the purpose of improving the patients' immune response. We have taken this approach, as a matter of policy, because the use of scarce blood component resources for such purposes in dying patients simply does not seem justified on medical or humanitarian grounds.

Antibiotics will be administered intravenously if a specific, treatable focus of infection can be identified and, hopefully, cultured. Triple therapy, if indicated, will not be withheld. Such situations must be distinguished, nevertheless, from the more common clinical presentation in which the patient becomes febrile, often in the range of 100°F–102°F, without any ascertainable focus of infection. The febrile response in these patients is often related to tumor necrosis and dehydration for which vigorous antibiotic therapy will serve no purpose.

Renal Failure

The problem of renal failure secondary to tumor encroachment upon the ureters is most conspicuous in the management of cervical carcinomas. The laterally spreading, aggressive cervical lesion quickly impinges on one, then both, ureters. Notwithstanding current pabulums, choices of one mode of death over another remain terrible choices. Concerning ureteral diversion to an ileal or other conduit, or the placement of a loop nephrostomy, it is our policy to discuss these surgical procedures with the patient or, if the patient is unwilling or unable to tolerate such discussion, with family members. It is our experience that, while ureteral diversion of one form or another has resulted in some slight prolongation of life, the quality of life for such patients in their final months has not been good. The heart pumps, the lungs exchange oxygen, the kidneys rid the body of metabolic waste, but the catabolic process continues unabated and the tumor grows without surcease. The patient becomes extraordinarily cachectic and ultimately dies, if not from sepsis, from cardiorespiratory failure. Pain relief becomes an almost insurmountable problem.

Progressive uremic poisoning from ureteral obstruction, on the other hand, probably means a somewhat more rapid demise, but with less pain and an arguably better passing. Tissue edema is, however, significant—and who is to say that the swollen, edematous visage of the dying patient in renal failure is to be preferred over the skeletal, tachycardic, tachypnic countenance of the nephrostomized patient. To the extent that we have a bias on this issue, it is probably in favor of avoiding additional surgical procedures and allowing renal failure to ensue.

Withdrawal or Withholding of Treatment

Controversy over such matters as the withdrawal or withholding of treatment, the issuance of NO CODE orders, the patient's right to die, and death with dignity has resulted in a plethora of articles, reviews, and commentaries in both medical and legal publications. From a practical, rather than a technical and legal point-of-view our situation in dealing with terminal gynecologic malignancy is rather more straightforward than terminal illness in medicine as a whole. There are several reasons for this. First, death secondary to gynecologic malignancy usually ensues as a result of hypovolemic shock, sepsis, uremic coma, or cardiorespiratory arrest. Rarely do we encounter the problems posed by mechanical ventilation, dialysis, intra-aortic balloon pumps or similar technological devices, which may support an otherwise mentally intact patient. Second, since the invasive aspect of our supportive care is often limited to intravenous lines, bladder catheters and nasogastric or intestinal tubes, patients rarely request discontinuance of these simple modalities. Third, in the final phases of the illness, as the malignancy takes its inexorable toll, the patient usually becomes comatose and thus legally incompetent to participate in decisions pertaining to the management of her subsequent care. Fourth, by definition, a terminal state associated with gynecologic malignancy does not involve the ambiguities which are associated with ascertaining diagnosis and prognosis in nonmalignant or even early malignant disease. Here we do not have to make judgments about maintaining the failing heart, lungs or kidneys while the patient's sensorium remains completely unaffected. Finally, we manage patients in a setting of minimal legal exposure. If the patient dies because supportive care was withdrawn or withheld, the claim ultimately reduces to the allegation that the patient would have lived some additional period of time had some treatment been effected or had some modality not been withheld. With a terminal malignancy, the actual time of death is impossible to predict and compensable damages in such claims are difficult, if not impossible, to assess and even more difficult to prove in court. Moreover, the opposite claim, that the patient was kept alive too long by supportive modalities and thus deprived of "death with dignity" is extraordinarily uncommon. Again these assessments are made in the context of gynecologic malignancies where terminal care is largely supportive and not highly invasive.

Although issues such as the withholding or withdrawal of resuscitative and/or life-sustaining procedures and equipment, the writing of NO CODE orders, refusal of treatment by the dying patient, and the attainment of "death with dignity" are interrelated, it is useful to separate them for purposes of analysis and for purposes of developing some general principles which will be applicable to the care of the terminal patient in most jurisdictions.

The concept that an individual shall have control over her person in obtaining medical care and shall have a right of determination in undertaking or refusing medical and surgical treatment is not by any means of recent origin. The criminal offense of battery, an unpermitted touching, expressed the idea that a citizen was to be free of violence to his or her person in a civilized society. In early decisions concerning claims of injury from surgical procedures to portions of the body other than those intended for treatment, courts resorted again to the idea of an unpermitted touching to find the defendant liable for his acts. Over the years it became apparent, however, that the criminal offense of battery was not properly applied in medical and surgical situations. The conduct of the physician or surgeon was not undertaken with the intent of doing harm to the patient as in the criminal context. What was really involved was medical negligence, a deviation from accepted standards of practice, for example, in operating on the wrong leg or in performing on patient "A" a procedure intended for patient "B". Such claims were cognizable in accordance with general tort principles of negligence. Claims arising out of a patient's not having agreed to the performance of a procedure or not having been adequately apprised of the risks and benefits of a procedure before agreeing to it presented issues of informed consent. The doctrine of informed consent is a reaffirmation that the patient is in control of the disposition of her person and that without informed consent, an intelligent, knowing disposition cannot be made.

A constitutional right respecting the individual's control over his or her person was found in the line of cases which legalized the sale of contraceptives in states forbidding such sale. This constitutional basis, is founded upon an unwritten right of privacy said to exist in the penumbra of specific guarantees of the Bill of Rights. This unwritten constitutional right of privacy is the basis upon which "death with dignity" really, refusal of treatment—and the related matters of the withholding or withdrawal of treatment are grounded.

With the foregoing as background, some general principles can be distilled. In general, most of the knotty problems in this area have involved the patient who is no longer mentally competent to participate meaningfully in decisions about her care as well as the competent patient who refuses treatment and who will, as a result of such refusal, probably die sooner. Legal competence implies that the patient understands the relative risks and alternatives which have been presented to her and her decision, therefore, reflects a deliberate, considered choice. One will appreciate that not only is the patient's competence or incompetence sometimes unclear, but the timing of the inquiry regarding competency and the use or non-use of particular drugs at that time can be manipulated so as to alter the outcome of the inquiry. Clearly the question of legal competency may become an issue unto itself. Notwithstanding the fact, there is no legal requirement which mandates a psychiatric consultation when competency is in question; moreover, attending gynecologists rarely, if ever, take the time to conduct a formal mental status examination in their daily assessment of the patient.

Assuming for purposes of discussion that competency or lack thereof can be determined in regard to a particular patient, the legalities are more straightforward. If the patient requests ordinary care, no legal issue or controversy is likely to arise. Extraordinary care in this context is most often referable to resuscitation in the event of cardiopulmonary arrest. It is clear that a competent patient may prospectively choose for herself the withholding of resuscitation or the withdrawal of a life-support system.

There are several lines of reasoning which have been used in formulating the legal justification for such a choice; three settings are illustrative: 1) the applicability of a Natural Death Act; 2) the refusal by the patient of lifesaving or supporting treatment, and 3) a terminal condition with death imminent.

A Natural Death Act, provides that the individual is allowed to decide under what circumstances and to what extent her life will be prolonged through the utilization or withholding of resuscitative and/or life-sustaining procedures and equipment. She does this by executing a document which directs withholding or withdrawal of such procedures or equipment if her condition is terminal and if death is imminent. The physician(s) and hospital are protected against civil and criminal liability if they comply with the patient's directive. This is an instance of compliance with the patient's wishes expressed through the mechanism of a written directive and a statutory procedure. Nevertheless, such statutes constitute evidence that legislatures are predisposed to allow the individual, usually on right-of-privacy grounds, to specify in advance the limits of medical care and treatment to which he or she will be subjected in a terminal illness.

The second setting is concerned with the competent patient who simply refuses, orally or in writing, life-saving or life-sustaining treatment. Specific facts may sometimes necessitate a balancing of the interests of the state vis-à-vis the individual's right to refuse such treatment, but in the case of the competent patient with a terminal gynecologic malignancy, the individual's right will almost always be upheld over the interest of the state. Coincidentally, the health care providers will be protected against potential claims of liability arising out of their implicit or explicit acceptance of the patient's refusal of treatment. One can appreciate that the balancing of the state's interest versus the individual's right may be more difficult where the patient is younger, where death is not imminent, and where third parties, such as minor children, are involved. Moreover, if one considers young patients with non-malignant and non-terminal conditions, as for example, life-threatening third trimester bleeding in a Jehovah's Witness patient, a very different result is likely to ensue as a result of the balancing of competing interests required under the law. A state interest has been found predominant to prevent suicide, to protect minor children, and to protect the desire of the medical profession to act affirmatively to preserve life. And where the state's interest is paramount, the physician may be found liable where he or she has abandoned treatment or ordered the withholding of treatment in accordance with the patient's expressed wish.

The third setting, again assuming a competent patient, is that which involves a terminal condition and imminent death. A slightly different verbal formulation refers to irreversibly and irreparably ill patients whose death is imminent. Imminent death is defined as death within two weeks. For purposes of comparison, such patients are said to be in roughly equivalent medical condition to those who, pursuant to the provisions of a Natural Death Act, have directed that treatment be withheld.

It is in cases such as these, as well as those involving incompetent patients, that the legal status of withholding resuscitation is most unclear. Several rationales have been offered in support of the legality of withholding treatment under these circumstances. First, most Natural Death Act legislation provides that, where death is imminent, a right to effect or withdraw life-saving treatment exists outside of the statute. This presumably refers to medical decisions made in accordance with accepted standards of medical practice by qualified physicians. Second, dicta in the *Karen Ann Quinlan* decision state that the general principles of the decision, which deals with withdrawal of life-support equipment, might be applicable to terminal cases other than withdrawal of life support. That is, such decisions are medical decisions best made by physicians without the intervention of the courts. Third, the rationale is offered that, inasmuch as no liability can accrue to the physician in the absence of a duty to act, and inasmuch as one's duty to act should be in reference to ordinary care, and inasmuch as CPR should be considered extraordinary care, there should be no liability where, in the exercise of reasonable medical judgment, resuscitative efforts have been withheld.

So, as to the competent patient with a terminal gynecologic malignancy, it is clear that she can direct the withdrawal or withholding of life-sustaining procedures or equipment. This may include her direction that orders-not-to-resuscitate be written by her attending physician. Contrariwise, such orders may *not* properly be written without the express consent, whether oral or written, of the competent patient.

One reason that dealing with the competent patient is more straightforward, from a medical-legal viewpoint, then dealing with the incompetent patient is the absence of a duty to deal with the patient's family except as a matter of courtesy and compassion. The physician-patient relationship does not involve third parties, although most patients will want a spouse, family member or close friend to be informed of her condition or prognosis. Quite often, however, we find that the patient expressly directs that her spouse and others *not* be told and, while we may attempt to convince her of the benefit of letting others know of her true condition, we are professionally bound to maintain her confidences and our knowledge of her case, if that is her desire. To make disclosures of confidential information against the express will of the patient would justify charges of professional wrongdoing although, from a realistic point-of-view, such charges rarely materialize because the prospective plaintiff, the patient, expires.

When dealing with the incompetent patient regarding issues of the withdrawal or withholding of life-sustaining equipment or procedures, the problem is more difficult. In such circumstances we communicate with the spouse or other family members in an attempt to assess what the patient's wishes might have been had she anticipated the present circumstances. We do not communicate with family for the purpose of ascertaining their wishes, *per se*, although family members doubtless suppose this to be the case. Many commentators have correctly made the point that the desires and interests of the family may not coincide with those of the patient. In the extreme case, family members may have reason to hope for an early demise while the comatose patient may have wished for a maximum medical effort to prolong life. More often, the family members, their motives tinged with guilt arising out of a sense that they have not done enough in the past, insist that everything possible, including resuscitation and ventilation support, be done to prolong life.

An occasional case report has given the impression that the attending physician caught in this situation is obliged to seek a court's decision before withholding or withdrawing life-sustaining equipment or procedures. This is clearly a minority view. Most courts which have examined the issue place the responsibility squarely upon the physician to treat the patient in accordance with accepted standards of practice and to make decisions pertaining thereto, including the withholding or withdrawing of life-sustaining equipment or procedures. While concurrence by family members with the proposed course of management is not required as a matter of law, it is generally worthwhile to involve them in the decision. Usually, the family will concur, or at least offer no opposition to, the proposed mode of management. Where the family of the incompetent patient does offer opposition to a proposed course involving withdrawal or withholding of life-sustaining equipment or procedures, the prudent course is to work through the legal system, usually with the appointment of a *guardian ad litem* for the dying patient and a court order directing or denying implementation of the proposed plan of management. The necessity for involving the legal system has arisen infrequently for the reasons cited at the beginning of this section.

Euthanasia

The AMA's House of Delegates adopted the following statement on euthanasia in 1973:

> The intentional termination of the life of one human being by another—mercy killing—is contrary to that for which the medical profession stands and is contrary to the policy of the American Medical Association. The cessation of the employment of extraordinary means to prolong the life of the body when there is irrefutable evidence that biological death is imminent is the decision of the patient/or his immediate family. The advice and judgment of the physician should be freely available to the patient and/or his immediate family.

Aid in dying pertains to an individual whose condition is leading irreversibly to death in the near future. Provocation of death, so-called "active" euthanasia, deliberately curtails life by artifically intervening in the vital processes that still subsist, in order to hasten death. In most countries active euthanasia is an intentional homicide, punishable under criminal law, even if done at the request of the patient.

What is believed to be the first plebiscite on active euthanasia was held in Switzerland in 1977. Voters of Zurich approved the initiation of legislation permitting doctors to perform euthanasia if requested by patients "suffering from an incurable, painful and definitely fatal disease."

"Passive" euthanasia, on the other hand, is the act of allowing a patient to die by renouncing measures that would prolong her life. It may involve omission or discontinuation of life supportive measures, but not renouncing those measures which add to the comfort of the patient.

The Cost of Dying

It is almost impossible to assess the cost of a terminal illness except in relationship to a specific patient. It is fair to say, however, that except in the case of sudden death the costs can be staggering, even if only maintenance care is provided. Eli Ginzberg of Columbia University recently provided an account of the last six months of his 93-year-old mother's life. Despite a cooperative physician who specialized in geriatric care and who made house-calls, the availability of relatively low-cost personnel to provide round-the-clock home nursing care, and a total of only 6 weeks' hospitalization out of the last six months of life, the aggregate cost of this woman's terminal illness of six months was $31,000. Two hospital admissions cost $15,000. Round-the-clock geriatric care was $10,000. Physician fees totaled $5,000. Ambulance, drugs, lab tests and miscellaneous items totaled $1,000. As Dr. Ginzberg asks in his account, "How do families with limited resources cope with such costs of dying?"

Numerous studies have compared the cost of terminal illness in hospitals as opposed to homes. One such study compared expenses of home care versus hospital care during the last two weeks of life of patients terminally ill with malignant disease. The hospital cost was reportedly 10.5 times greater than the home cost, due principally to the quantity of diagnostic and therapeutic services and ancillary personnel provided for hospitalized patients. Although such services as radiology, radiotherapy, physical therapy and respiratory therapy provided examples of costs which were significant and which had no counterpart in home care, the most significant single item of all expenses remained the hospital room. In the study cited, costs for 19 hospitalized patients exceeded costs for 19 matched patients cared for at home by $106,000. These data were obtained in the Philadelphia area during 1979.

As any physician regularly involved with terminal patients knows, it is often difficult to persuade consultant physicians, housestaff, technical specialists (respiratory therapists, physiotherapists, etc.), and others to desist in ordering or actually executing tests and treatment inappropriate to a patient's terminal status. Many cases do not warrant even a repeat CBC, let along IPPB treatments, CT scans, and other tests and services. In the face of all of this, it is clear that there are substantial economic pressures to care for terminal patients outside of the hospital. These pressures will continue to mount despite practical problems associated with home care for patients with gynecologic malignancy, not the least of which is the problem of acute and chronic hemorrhage.

Hospital and Hospice

The concept of hospice, a place of shelter and comfort for one departing this life, has received a good deal of public attention over the last decade or so. Dr. Cicely Saunders opened St. Christopher's Hospice in Sydenham, London, in 1968. Basically, hospices are organized to provide complete care for the dying patient including physical care, emotional care and social care. For the hospice to function well, a high ratio of staff to patients is required. The best-known and most successful hospice programs are in institutions which are able to rely on large numbers of volunteers in addition to the full-time staff.

It is beyond the scope of this chapter to discuss hospice philosophy, the establishment of hospice programs, the most commonly encountered problems in setting up a hospice, and other issues pertaining to hospice care. We do wish to convey, nevertheless, several practical problems which we have encountered in relation to both hospice care and home care of the patient with a terminal gynecologic malignancy. First, it should be obvious that hospice care becomes appropriate only after the decision has been made to abandon all therapeutic modalities such as hyperalimentation, intravenous fluids, blood or blood component transfusion, and intravenous antibiotics to name but a few. If the patient or patient's family feel that the days, weeks or perhaps months of additional life which might be gained from such treatment ought to be sought, hospice care will not suffice. Second, while it is often said that terminal patients would prefer to die in a hospice or home surroundings rather than in the hospital, our experience has been somewhat to the contrary. Most patients with terminal gynecologic malignancies have been hospitalized on multiple occasions in the final twelve months of their illness. They are, more often than not, very familiar and very comfortable in the hospital at which they have been receiving ongoing care. They know the atmosphere, the routine and most important, the nurses and staff. They often report anxiety-provoking experiences in connection with attempts at care by unfamiliar physicians and staff in unfamiliar institutions. Third, patients with terminal gynecologic malignancies unfortunately often present with bowel obstruction and/or hemorrhage. While bowel obstruction and progressive secondary inanition can perhaps be allowed to take its toll in the hospice, acute hemorrhage is not something most hospices care to deal with (unless one is speaking simply of an agonal event). These patients are usually best managed in a hospital. Fourth, while we would like to believe that there are sufficient numbers of willing family physicians, general internists, referring gynecologists, and other primary care practitioners to care for the terminal patient at home or in a convenient hospice facility, our experience has been that such practitioners do not want to deal with the terminal care of these patients. Whether or not a request to such physicians for terminal care is regarded as "dumping" the patient, we do not know. We do know that most referring physicians, whether gynecologists, family physicians, general internists, or others are unhappy when we return to them for terminal care a patient we have been managing for the past two, three or more years.

Our concept is that a hospital can serve as a hospice. We feel that a nurse-conducted primary care unit for terminal patients can exist within the administrative structure of a large community or university hospital. Such an arrangement potentially affords the patient the best of both worlds with a maximum opportunity for coordination of the therapeutic and/or palliative effort in the most effective way. This should be our goal coupled with an earnest attempt to keep the patient in her home setting for the maximum allowable time.

Priorities for Future Terminal Care

Planning of future methods and facilities for care of the terminal patient should begin now. In 1984 we are faced with huge federal budget deficits combined with decreased spending for delivery of health care. Parallel problems exist on the state and local level. Pressures continue to build in the U.S. to decrease the total cost for health care of all types. It is not reasonable to assume that there will be a great increase in the construction of new hospice facilities or any type of facility devoted primarily to the care of the terminal patient.

Several general observation suggest our future course. The most significant single factor in providing excellent terminal care is the availability of high-quality nursing. Doctors, social workers, physiotherapists, occupational therapists and others are important, but those who provide nursing care at all levels—registered nurse, licensed practical nurse, nurse's aid—are most important.

The second most important factor is the relief of severe intractable pain. This issue has been addressed previously.

Third, care at home, under the supervision of a physician and with the support of a nursing team, is undoubtedly the very best terminal care when successful.

Fourth, the success of the hospice movement is due to the skill and commitment of the paid staff and the excellent volunteer support such units have received.

Fifth, the training and education of nurses, doctors and other health care providers in the rendering of terminal care is far more important than promoting a large increase in hospices.

Sixth, the population concentration in major cities poses completely insurmountable problems to providing good terminal care if the issue is addressed in terms of providing specialized facilities.

What direction, therefore, is appropriate in establishing priorities for terminal care in the future? It is our feeling, as in the British experience, that shortages of trained staff and insufficient funds argue conclusively against any attempt to develop more specialist units for terminal care. Emphasis must be upon the *dissemination of principles of terminal care throughout the health care system.* The community hospital has the most important role to play, both in providing traditional in-patient services and as the base from which and in which nurse-conducted, physician-supervised, primary care for terminal patients may be given. Such nursing care services must be available throughout the community to maximize opportunities for home care. This approach, we believe, will result in high-quality terminal care within the framework of health care delivery which is already in existence. Not only will such an approach involve lower levels of designated funding but, more important, will be susceptible to more rapid implementation. Continuing efforts to educate doctors, nurses and others members of the health care team about the medical, psychological and social aspects of dying and bereavement are implicit in all of the foregoing.

Conclusions

Sir William Temple, three centuries ago, said "In all diseases of the body or mind, it is happy to have an able physician for a friend, or a discreet friend for a physician." The care and treatment of the dying depends ultimately upon the physician's appreciation of his own patient's personality. Such an appreciation truly involves the art of medicine, an art which may be rapidly vanishing. In the practice of this art, it often matters less what medicine is given than what we give of ourselves along with our medicines.

Most patients have the feeling that death is near. Some know it well enough, yet want nothing said about it. Or perhaps, while they like to talk of it with the doctor and nurses, they cannot bear to speak of it to their families. Some families, on the other hand, prefer not to be told the truth and are particularly anxious that nothing be said to alarm the patient. In other cases, perfect frankness all around is wanted. This may be of comfort to the family at the time or later in retrospect. Much of the uncertainty of what should be said or unsaid is generally related to unawareness that death is almost always preceded by a degree of willingness to die. The acceptance of approaching death is its natural accompaniment.

Human nature is such that uncertainty is probably the hardest emotion to bear. What we don't know, we fear the most, and therefore adds much to the distress of the family. However, if the family has been properly counseled, certain knowledge does ease the inevitable outcome.

INDEX

Numerals in *italics* indicate a figure, "t" following a page number indicates tabular material.

Abdomen, palpation of, 1
Adenocarcinoma, endometrial, adeno-
    matous hyperplasia and, 80
  tissue samples from D&C in, 98–99
Adrenal steroids, production of, in aging,
    36
Age of patient, as factor in cancer risk, 65
  as factor in repair of pelvic support, 153
  visiting gynecologist, 8
Aging, estrone production in, 36
  nutrition and, 12
Alcoholism, nutrition and, 15
Analgesia, for dying patient, 168–170
Androgen(s), secretion of, perimeno-
    pausal, 35
  therapy, in menopause, 44
Androstenedione, in premenopausal and
    menopausal women, 35
Anemia, of malignant disease, manage-
    ment of, 175
Anesthesia, examination under, in post-
    menopausal bleeding, 95–96
Anosmia, 12
Antibiotic treatment, for dying patient,
    176
Anticholinergic drugs, in urinary
    incontinence, 110
Anxiety, changes in eating habits in, 15
Ascites, in dying patient, treatment of,
    174

Back, exercise program, for osteoporosis
    patients, *29*
  pain, low, exercises for, 28, *30*
Back stretch exercise, *25*
Bicycle, stationary, 27
Biopsy, endometrial, 5–6
  for histologic diagnosis, in post-
    menopausal bleeding, 94

  in lesions of vulva, 7
  punch, in invasive cervical cancer,
    97–98
  in lichen sclerosus, 58–59
Bladder, capacity, and old age, 109–110
Bleeding, following posterior
    colpoperineoplasty, 129–130
  pelvic, in dying patient, management
    of, 171
  postmenopausal, 75–107
    as sign of neoplastic disease, 75, 103
    definition of, 77, 93
    diagnostic techniques in, 103
    differential diagnosis of, 83–92
    management of, 92–101
    nondefinitive findings in, 100–101
    follow-up in, 101–103
    sources of, 86–87t
Blood count, importance of, 7
Bone(s), loss, calcium intake and, 18
  strength, maintenance of, 11–12, 23
Bowel obstruction, in dying patient,
    management of, 172–173
Breast, cancer, estrogen therapy and,
    37–38
  carcinoma of, 47–54
    age incidence of, 48, *49*
    attitude of geriatric patient toward,
      52–53
    diagnosis of, 3
    in elderly, as unique problem, 53–54
    incidence of, 47
    staging of, 51–52
    surgery in, in aged, 48–51
    treatment of, results of, 52
  examination of, explanation of, to
    patient, 3
  mammography in, 3, 53
  procedure for, by physician, 2–3
  self, 3–4, *2-3*

Breast (*continued*)
    in total evaluation, 2-4
    "towel trick" for, 53
    nodulation of, evaluation of, 2-3

Calcium, foods high in, 18, 19-20t
    intake, of American women, 18
        measures to increase, 22
    needs, throughout life, 18
    -rich diet, 18
Calorie(s), distribution, for older women, 17
    needs, for older adults, 17
Cancer(s), diagnosis of, 66
        during D&C, 99-100
    estrogen and, 36-38
    past history of, endometrial carcinoma and, 82
    preoperative evaluation in, 67-68
    risk of developing, age and race factors influencing, 65
        with aging, 65
    screening for, 66
    specific, management of, 68-73
    treatment of, 66
    See also specific sites of cancer
Carbohydrates, complex, in diet, 17
Carcinoma *in situ*, endometrial, 80
Carcinoma(s), of breast. *See* Breast, carcinoma of
    gynecologic, problems in patients dying from, 168, 177
Cardiovascular system, exercise and, 23
Caruncles, urethral, 112
Cervix, cancer of, Pap tests and, 7
        postmenopausal bleeding and, 75
        risk factors for development of, 65
        treatment of, 66, 70
    lesions, evaluation of, 5
        postmenopausal bleeding in, 83-84
Chemotherapy, for elderly, 68
    following resection of ovarian cancer, 72
    nutrition and, 14
Collagenolysis, estrogen and, osteoporosis related to, 40
Colon, aging and, nutrition and, 13-14
    involvement of, in ovarian carcinoma, 72
Colpocleisis, Le Fort, 113
Colpoperineoplasty (posterior), age of patients for, 118-119
    associated operative procedures and, 128
    complications of, 129-130

follow-up in, 128-129
    incidence of need for, 118
    painful dyspareunia following, 120
    parity and, 118
    results of, 129-132
    techniques of, dissection in, 120-124, *121, 122, 123, 124*
        preparation for, 120, 129
        suturing in, 125-128, *126, 127*
    techniques of obstetric deliveries and, 119, 119t
Colpopexy, in prolapse of post-hysterectomy vagina, 163-164
Colposcopy, in assessment of postmenopausal bleeding, 94
Communication, as important, 4, 9
    with dying patient, 178-182, 188
    with family of dying patient, 182
Conization, surgical, of cervix, in abnormal Pap smears, 97, 98
Constipation, definition of, 14
Contraceptive medications, endometrial carcinoma and, 81
Copper, needs, of elderly, 21
Curettage, uterine, in postmenopausal bleeding, 98-100
Curette(s), for endometrial biopsy, 5-6, *6*

D&C, in postmenopausal bleeding, 98-100
    precautions in perforation during, 100
Death, management of, 165
"Death with dignity," 165, 178, 179
Dehydration, correction of, in dying patient, 171-172
Dentures, taste and, 12
Depression, changes in eating habits in, 15
Detrusor dyssynergia, urinary incontinence in, 110-111
Diagnostic studies, in gynecologic cancer, 67
Disabled, exercise for, 28
Discharges, documentation of, in history, 1
Diuretics, and urinary incontinence, 110
Drug(s), conditions caused by, 14
    contraceptive, endometrial carcinoma and, 81
    for dying patient, 169-170
    reducing saliva, 13
    taste and, 12
    therapies, evaluation of, in urinary incontinence, 111
    use of by elderly, 14

Dying, cost of, 183–184
  process of, as progressive, 165–166
Dying patient, ascites and paracentesis
    in, 174–175
  bowel obstruction in, 172–173
  care of, 165–188
    continuum of, 167–168
    regimens in, 165
  chronic anemia in, 175
  dehydration and electrolyte imbalance
    in, 171–172
  future terminal care for, priorities for,
    186–187
  hyperalimentation of, 166, 173–174
  immune suppression and antibiotic
    treatment for, 175–176
  pain and analgesia in, 168–170
  pelvic hemorrhage in, 170–171
  physician and, 187–188
  renal failure in, 176–177
  withdrawal or withholding treatment
    from, 177–183
Dysosmia, 12
Dyspareunia, painful, following
    colpoperineoplasty, 120
Dystrophy, in lichen sclerosus, 57
  mixed, 57

Elderly, definition of, 48, 109
  See also Geriatric patient(s)
Electrolyte imbalance, correction of, in
    dying patient, 171
Embolization, of pelvic vessels, of dying
    patient, 171
Endocervix, dilation of, technique for, 99
Endocrinology, of menopause, 75–78
  of perimenopausal years, 34–36
Endometrial biopsy, 5–6
Endometrial polyps, 85–88
Endometrial screening, in postmeno-
    pausal bleeding, 94–95
Endometritis, 90–91
Endometrium, carcinoma of, estrogen
    therapy and, 37
  prognosis in, age as influence on, 70
  risk factors for development of, 65,
    80–83
  treatment of, 70–71, 71t
  tumor differentiation in, and prog-
    nosis in, 88
  hyperplasia, and adenocarcinoma, 80
  "nonphasic," 89–90
  postmenopausal, 78–80
Enterocele, grading of, 138–139
Epinephrine, for endometrial biopsy, 6

Episiotomy(ies), median, 116
  mediolateral, 116–117, 131
Esophagus, dysmotility of, nutrition in,
    13
Estrogen(s), deficiency, 33.45
  as factor in repair of pelvic
    support, 154
  physiologic changes incidental to,
    112–114
  exogenous, and endometrial car-
    cinoma, 81–82, 88, 90t
  endometrial polyps and, 88
  postmenopausal bleeding and, 85,
    89–90, 90t, 101
  production, postmenopausal, 36, 77, 78
Estrogen therapy, administration of
    progestogens with, 101–102
  and cancer, 7, 36–38
  in estrogen deficiency-related
    problems, 112–113
  for geriatric patients, 9
  management of, 42–44
  and osteoporosis, 36–42
  postmenopausal, hip fracture and,
    39–40
  seeking of, 33
Estrone, in premenopausal and post-
    menopausal women, 35–36, 77
Estrone sulfate, in estrogen replacement
    therapy, 43
Ethylestradiol, in bone loss, 39
Euthanasia, 183
  "passive," 183
Evaluation, of total woman, 1–9
Examination(s), gynecologic,
    importance of regular, 7–8
  procedures in, 1–7
  under anesthesia, in postmeno-
    pausal bleeding, 95–96
Exercise(s), benefits of, 22–24
  climbing-the-wall, 25
  continuing of, 11
  for disabled, 28
  extension, resisted, 26
  fitness and, 24
  flexion, resisted, 26
  guidelines, for beginners, 28–31
  history, taking of, 23–24
  interest and motivation for, 31
  lack of, hazards of, 11
  in low back pain, 30
  medical examination prior to
    planning, 24
  pendular, 25
  recommendations for, 12, 24
  regimen, for osteoporosis patients, 29

Exercise(s) (*continued*)
  regular, weight reduction with, 23
  rotation, resisted, *26*
  shoulder shrug, *25*
  side-bend, resisted, *26*
  specific, for specific problems, 27-28
  types of, for older patients, 24-27
  upper back stretch, *25*
Exercise equipment, 28
Exercise facilities, 28

Fallopian tube, cancer of, 91
Fat(s), dietary, need for, 17
  intake, reducing of, 22
Fiber, daily requirements of, 21
  sources of, 21-22
Financial factors, influencing nutrition,
    15-16
Fitness, exercise and, 24
Fluorine, importance of, 21
  toxicity of, 21
Follicle stimulating hormone (FSH),
    circulating, in perimenopause,
    34-35
  postmenopausal plasma levels of,
    77-78, *79*
Fracture(s), hip, incidence of, 38-39
  postmenopausal estrogen use and,
    39-40

Gastrointestinal tract, exercise and, 23
  nutrition and, 13-14
Genital tract, lower, postmenopausal
    bleeding from, 83
Geriatric patient(s), bleeding in, 8
  breast examination for, 8
  carcinoma in, 8
  complaints of, 8
  exercise for, 24-27
  incidence of, in U.S., 135
Geriatrics, definition of, 47
Glossdynia, 13
Glosspyrexia, 13
Golf, as exercise, 27
Gynecologist, age of patients visiting, 8

Half-way Grading System (HWGS), for
    repair of pelvic support, *137*,
    138-140, *139, 141*, 155-156
Healing, nutrition and, 16-17
Hemorrhage. *See* Bleeding
Hemorrhoids, in rectocele, 120
Hip, fracture of, incidence of, 38-39
  postmenopausal estrogen use and,
    39-40

joints, immobility of, as factor in repair
    of pelvic support, 154
History taking, importance of, 1-2
Holding, loss of pelvic support and, *139*,
    140, 143-144
Hormone(s), and cancer, 7
  for geriatric patients, 9
  ovarian, acyclic, and endometrial car-
    cinoma, 81
  postmenopausal, 77-78, *78*
  response, ovarian cycle and, 76-77, *76*
  thyroid, treatment with, endometrial
    cancer and, 82-83
Hospice, care of terminal patients in, 185
Hospital, dying patient in, 185-186
Hostility, changes in eating habits in, 15
Hyperalimentation, of dying patient,
    166, 173-174
Hyperplasia(s), endometrial, following
    menopause, 80
  postmenopausal bleeding in, 85
Hyposmia, 12
Hysterectomy, colpoperineoplasty fol-
    lowing, 124
  in endometrial carcinoma, 70
  in postmenopausal bleeding, 101
  vaginal, procedures replaced by,
    159-160

Illness, chronic, nutrition and, 14
Immune suppression, in malignant
    disease, 175-176
Immunologic defenses, nutrition and,
    16-17
Incontinence, urinary, grading, *139*, 140
  stress, 109, 110, 111
Informed consent, 178-179
Infusion pump, continuous, for dying
    patient, 169-170
Intestine, small, absorption in, nutrition
    and, 13
  cell proliferation in, nutrition and, 13
Iron, needs of elderly, 21

Jogging, stationary, 27

Kyphosis, 28

Labia, adhesions of, 112-113
Lactalase, 22
Laxative abuse, 14
LeFort colpocleisis, 113
Light, for dying patient, 166-167
Luteinizing hormone (LH), increase in
    circulating, 34-35

postmenopausal plasma levels of, 77-78, *79*
Libido, factors influencing, 34
Lichen sclerosus, 55
  alcohol injection in, 60
  immunologic theories of, 60
  histopathological criteria for, 56, *56*
  hormones deficiencies in, 60
  management of, 58-60
  perivulvar-perianal neurotomy procedures in, 60
  progesterone therapy in, 60
  punch biopsy in, 57-58
  symptoms of, 56-57, *57*
  synonyms for, 55-56
  testosterone preparation in, 59
Life expectancy, of American female, 47t

Magnesium, deficiencies, conditions causing, 18-21
  needs, of elderly, 18
Malnutrition, causes of, 16
  tests to detect, 16
  treatment of, 11
  typical patient with, 11
Mammography, 3, 53
Manchester-Fothergill operation, 160
Marshall-Marchetti-Krantz operation, 162
Mastectomy, modified radical, for geriatric patient, 50
  simple, for geriatric patient, 50-51
Meals, to improve nutrition, 22
Megavitamin quackery, 17
Menopause, beginning of, signs of, 77, 92
  endocrinology of, 75-78
  estrogen therapy in. *See* Estrogen therapy
  reactions to, 33
  therapies in, alternate, 43-44
  See also Perimenopause; Postmenopause
Menstruation, documentation of, in history, 1
  unusual patterns of, investigation of, 92-93
Mental health, exercise and, 23
Mineral needs, of elderly, 18-22
Monitoring, invasive, during surgery for elderly, 67
Morphine sulfate, for dying patient, 169, 170
Motivation, for exercise, 31
Mouth, of dying patient, care of, 166
Mucosa, urethral, prolapse of, 112

Musculoskeletal system, exercise and, 23

Natural Death Act, 180-181
Needle aspiration, in breast mass, 3
Nipple, examination of, by physician, 2
  self, 4
Nutrition, aging and, 12
  alcohol and, 15
  assessment of, 16
  chemotherapy and, 14
  in chronic illness, 14
  diseases affecting, 12-14
  drug use and, 14
  gastrointestinal factors influencing, 13-14
  good, importance of, 11
  healing and, 16
  immunologic defenses and, 16
  improvement of, suggestions for, 22
  income influencing, 15-16
  needs, of elderly, 16-17
  oral cavity disease and, 12-13
  physiologic changes affecting, 12-14
  psychological factors influencing, 15
  radiation therapy and, 14
  social problems affecting, 15-16
  surgery and, 14
  taste and smell influencing, 12
  tobacco use and, 15

Obesity, as cause of malnutrition, 12
  avoiding of, suggestions for, 22
  development of, 12
  endometrial cancer and, 82
  and estrone production, 36
Oncology, geriatric gynecologic, 65-73
Oral cavity, disease of, nutrition and, 12
Oral hygiene, good, importance of, 13
Osteoporosis, back exercise regimen for, *29*
  conditions caused by, 38
  definition of, 38
  diagnosis of, 40
  estrogens and, 38-41
  exercise and, 11, 23
  factors influencing development of, 41
  in men and women, compared, 38
  postmenopausal, 38, 39
  and slender body habitus, 40-41
Outpatient examination, in postmenopausal bleeding, 93
Ovarian cycle, and hormonal response, 76-77, *76*
Ovarian hormones, acyclic, and endometrial carcinoma, 81

Ovary(ies), cancer of, abnormal genital
    bleeding in, 91
    involvement of colon in, 72
    postmenopausal bleeding in, 91-92
    risk factors for development of, 65
    surgical technique in, 72
    treatment of, 66, 71
Oxygen demand, exercise and, 24

Pain, documentation of, in history, 1
    of dying patient, relief of, 168-170
Palpation, abdominal, 1, 4
    importance of, 4-5
    of lower extremities, 4
    of vagina, 5
Papanicolaou (Pap) smear, abnormal,
        histologic
    diagnosis in, 96-98
    in breast secretions, 2-3
    during estrogen replacement therapy,
        42
    in postmenopausal bleeding, 93-94
        as lacking significance, 102
    reasons for doing, 7
    value of, 102-103
Paracentesis, in ascites in dying patient,
        174-175
Parkinson's disease, 14
Patients, age of, going to gynecologist, 8
Pelvis, defects of, diagnosis of, *137, 139,*
        143-144
    evaluation of, 4
    functional supportive anatomy of, *141,*
        142-143
    loss of support of, causes of, 136-138
        definition of, 136
        grading system in, *137*, 138-142, *139*
        management of, 135-136, 144-153
            non-surgical, 144-145
            operative, 146-148, 147, 149, 150
            preoperative, 145-146
            problems, pitfalls, and solutions
                in, 153-155
            reparative concepts in, 148
            review of results of, 148-153, 151t,
                152t, 153t
            summary and conclusions on,
                155-157
        sites of, 136
        symptoms of, 136
Perimenopause, endocrinology of, 34-36
Perineum, care of, during vaginal
        delivery, 117-118
    lacerations of, causes of, 115-116, 118
        fissuring following, 120
        grading of, *137*, 138

incidence of, 118-119
    prevention of, 116-118, *117*, 119-120
    surgical management of. *See*
        Colpoperineoplasty (posterior)
    "washboard," following colpoperineo-
        plasty, 120
Pessary, vaginal, in pelvic support loss,
        145
    in uterovaginal prolapse, 113-114
Phosphorus needs, of elderly, 21
Physiologic abnormalities, correction of,
        before surgery, 68
Polycystic ovary syndrome, 81
Polyps, endometrial, 85-88
    adenomyomatous, 85
    functional, 85
    hyperplastic, 85
    search for, during D&C, 100
Position, change of, for dying patient,
        166
Postmenopausal bleeding. *See* Bleeding,
        postmenopausal
Postmenopause, sexuality in, 34
Postoperative care, of elderly, 50
Potassium needs, of elderly, 18
Preoperative evaluation, in cancer, 67
Progesterone, in estrogen replacement
        therapy, 43
    in lichen sclerosus, 60
Progestins, in menopause, 44
Progestogen(s), and osteoporosis, 38
    superimposed, in estrogen therapy,
        101-102
Progestogen challenge test, 37, 101-102
Protein requirements, 17
Psychological factors, influencing
        nutrition, 15
Pubococcygeal "holding," 144
Punch biopsy, in lichen sclerosus, 58

Quackery, megavitamin, 17

Race, as factor in cancer risk, 65
Racquet sports, as exercise, 27
Radiation therapy, contraindications to,
        68
    in endometrial carcinoma, 70-71
    following mastectomy, 50, 52
    nutrition and, 14
Rectocele, causes of, 115-116, 118, 131
    checking for, 131, *131*
    incidence of, 118
    prevention of, 116-118, *117*, 119-120
    surgical management of. *See*
        Colpoperineoplasty (posterior)
Rectovaginal examination, 6

Rectum, descent of, grading of, *137*, 138
  laceration of, increasing incidence of,
    130-131
Renal failure, in dying patient, management of, 176-177
Resuscitation, choice of, legal justification for, 179-181 Retropubic
  urethropexy, in urinary incontinence, 112

Saliva, loss of, nutrition and, 13
Salpingo-oophorectomy, in endometrial
  carcinoma, 70
Salt intake, reduction of, 22
Sarcomas, postmenopausal bleeding in,
  91
Schiller staining technique, 5
Sexual activity, during menopause, 34
Sexuality, human, 33-34
Shoulder shrug exercise, *25*
Skiing, as exercise, 27
Sleep, exercise and, 23
Slender body habitus, osteoporosis and,
  40-41
Social problems, influencing nutrition,
  15-16
Speculum, for vaginal inspection, 5
Staging of breast cancer, 51-52
Staining technique, Schiller, 5
Straining, loss of pelvic support and,
  136-138, *137*, 143-144
Stress urinary incontinence, 109, 110,
  111
"Stressless stress," 144-145
Surgery, in geriatric patient, factors
  influencing, 49-50
  nutrition and, 14
Swimming, as exercise, 27

Taste acuity, nutrition and, 12
Terminal care. *See* Dying patient
Testosterone, compounding of, for ointment preparation, 59
  secretion, premenopausal and menopausal, 35
  therapy, in lichen sclerosus, 58-59
Thyroid hormone, production, with aging,
  36
  treatment with, endometrial cancer
    and, 82-83
TNM system of cancer staging, 51-52
Tobacco use, diseases associated with, 15
Toluidine blue test, in lichen sclerosus, 58
Tongue, lesions of, nutrition and, 13
Tooth (teeth), loss of, 13
  nutrition and, 12-13

Thorax, of dying patient, "dilation" of,
  166
"Towel trick," for breast examination, 53

Uremic poisoning, in dying patient,
  176-177
Urethritis, estrogen therapy in, 43
Urethrocystoscopy, in pelvic support
  loss, 145
Urethropexy, retropubic, in urinary
  incontinence, 112
Urethrovesical problems, 109-114
Urinary incontinence, stress, 109, 110,
  111
Urine, control, difficulties in, 110-112
  evaluation of, at physical examination, 7
  value, residual, 110
Urodynamic studies, in pelvic support
  loss, 145
Uterine tube, cancer of, 91
Uterovaginal prolapse, 113
Uterus, as source of postmenopausal
  bleeding, 84-85
  curettage of, in postmenopausal bleeding, 98-100
  prolapse of, 160

Vagina, cancer of, after hysterectomy,
  treatment of, 69
  invasive, treatment of, 69-70
  risk factors associated with, 65
  treatment of, 66
  evaluation of, cellular evaluation in, 5
  technique for, 5
  length of, following repair of pelvic
    support, 155
  palpation of, 5
  posterior, relaxations and lacerations
    of, treatment of, 115-133
  post-hysterectomy prolapse of, classification of, 162
  diagnosis of, 161
  management of, 159-164
  preservation of sexual function in,
    159
  treatment of, 161-162
  Type I, repair of, 162-163
  Type II, repair of, 163-164
  rectovaginal examination of, 6
  secretions of, evaluation of, 5
Vaginitis, estrogen therapy in, 43
Vitamin D, 17
Vitamin(s), deficiency(ies), causes of, 17
  vitamins implicated in, 17
  needs, of elderly, 17

Vitamin(s) (*continued*)
  supplementation, 17
Vulva, aging, 55-63
  cancer of, associated conditions in, 68
    risk factors associated with, 65
    treatment of, 69
  disorders of, with aging, 61-62
  examination of, 7
  in lichen sclerosus. *See* Lichen sclerosus
    sus pruritus of, 55
  skin of, in aging, 55
Vulvectomy, in vulvar carcinoma, 69

Walking, as good exercise, 27
Water, daily requirements of, 21
  function of, in body, 21
Weight reduction, exercise for, 23
Woman, life expectancy of, 47t
  total, evaluation of, 1-9

Xerostomia, 13
Xylocaine, for biopsy, 6

Zinc, needs, of elderly, 21